BBS LONG & STRO

STRETCHING + FLEXIBILITY USING THE *BODY BEFORE SKILL*™ TRAINING METHOD

by Jessica Zoo

YOUR L&S ACCESS CODE FOR BBS ONLINE STUDIO:

Amazon2668L&S

LEGAL COPYRIGHT.   © Jessica Zoo Ltd 2020   www.BodyBeforeSkill.com

Second Edition | BODY BEFORE SKILL™ Training Method
Published by Jessica Zoo Ltd
Company registered in England 06634124
Parkshot House, 5 Kew Road, Richmond TW9 2PR

No portion of this book may be reproduced or distributed in any form without permission from Jessica Zoo Ltd, (trading as CheerConditioning.Academy and BODY BEFORE SKILL™ Training Method) as per U.K. copyright law and all other applicable international, federal, state and local laws, with ALL rights reserved.

PHOTOGRAPHY by Henk Oets and Juliano Grimaldi
DESIGNS by Jessica Zoo

HEALTH DISCLAIMER

THE INFORMATION SHARED IN THIS GUIDE AND ALL SUPPORTING MATERIALS ARE DESIGNED TO PROVIDE HELPFUL INSIGHTS INTO THE SUBJECTS DISCUSSED. THIS BOOK IS NOT MEANT TO BE USED, NOR SHOULD IT BE USED AS A REPLACEMENT FOR PROFESSIONAL COACHING OR FITNESS INSTRUCTION. IN THE CASE OF A NEED FOR ANY SUCH EXPERTISE CONSULT WITH THE APPROPRIATE PROFESSIONAL.

THIS BOOK DOES NOT CONTAIN ALL INFORMATION AVAILABLE ON THE SUBJECT. THIS GUIDE AND ALL SUPPORTING MATERIALS HAVE NOT BEEN CREATED TO BE SPECIFIC TO ANY INDIVIDUAL OR ORGANISATIONAL SITUATIONS OR NEEDS. EVERY EFFORT HAS BEEN MADE TO MAKE THIS GUIDE AND ALL SUPPORTING MATERIALS AS ACCURATE AS POSSIBLE. THERE MAY, HOWEVER, BE TYPOGRAPHICAL AND/OR CONTENT ERRORS. THEREFORE, THEY SHOULD SERVE ONLY AS A GENERAL GUIDE AND NOT AS THE ULTIMATE SOURCE OF SUBJECT INFORMATION.

REFERENCES ARE PROVIDED FOR INFORMATIONAL PURPOSES ONLY AND DO NOT CONSTITUTE ENDORSEMENT OF ANY WEBSITE OR ANY OTHER SOURCES. THE AUTHOR AND PUBLISHER SHALL HAVE NO LIABILITY OR RESPONSIBILITY TO ANY PERSON OR ENTITY REGARDING ANY LOSS OR DAMAGE INCURRED, DIRECTLY OR INDIRECTLY, BY THE INFORMATION CONTAINED IN THIS GUIDE AND ALL SUPPORTING MATERIALS.

To all the brilliant people who have been a part of the BODY BEFORE SKILL journey: past, present and future.

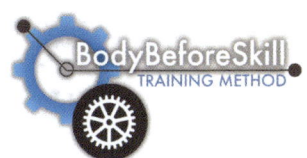

TABLE OF CONTENTS
BBS LONG & STRONG

INTRODUCTION..2
1. WHAT IS FLEXIBILITY.................................5
2. STRETCH TECHNIQUE..............................13
3. BODY STRETCHES....................................19
4. MYOFASCIAL RELEASE............................43
5. TRAINING PROGRAMS............................47
6. ONLINE WORKOUTS................................53

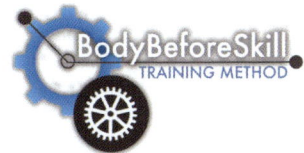

INTRODUCTION

Welcome and thank you for joining me on this BODY BEFORE SKILL™ flexibility journey. Let me tell you a little bit about what to expect from this guide and the BBS Online Studio workouts.

Since 2009, I have been pursuing the link between fitness, human movement and athletic performance through the sport of cheerleading. BODY BEFORE SKILL™ started as a simple mission: train the body first, the skills will follow. Train smarter, not harder, and reduce injuries.

The mission was dedicated to uncovering the mysteries of human performance: soaking in knowledge from a variety of disciplines: from cheerleading, gymnastics, dance, pilates, barre, yoga, martial arts, exercise to music, strength training, biokinetics and sports science. Throughout this journey, I realised:

- The human body is AMAZING: it can transform at any point in our lives with the right training and understanding.
- We never stop learning; knowledge is key to growth.
- Flexibility is a tough nut to crack: you need to understand how it works and use correct technique to see injury-free results!

After a few years hiatus from fitness, I had two very unexpected incidents that marked a fresh new start for me. In the one year that followed, through this approach I was able to reach new undiscovered limits of ability and flexibility and started to develop the BODY BEFORE SKILL™ Training Method.

Over 10 years, the method has evolved to combining the love of movement, sports science and the joy of music.

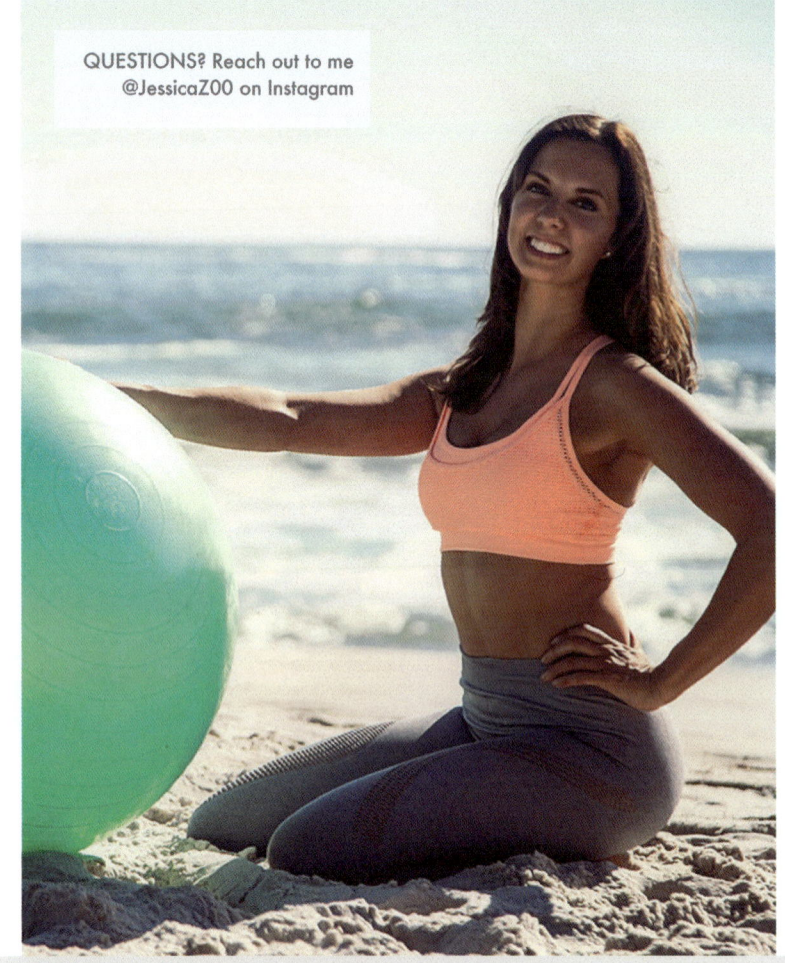

QUESTIONS? Reach out to me @JessicaZOO on Instagram

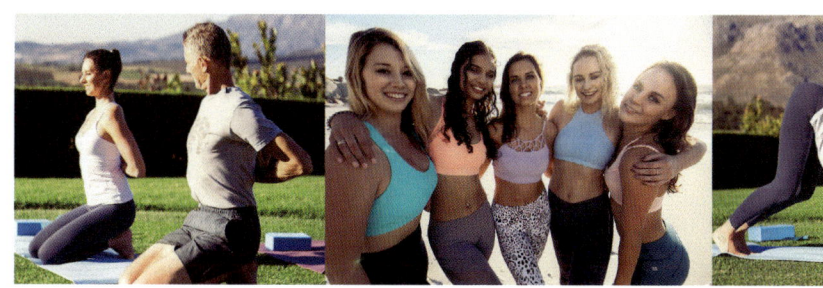
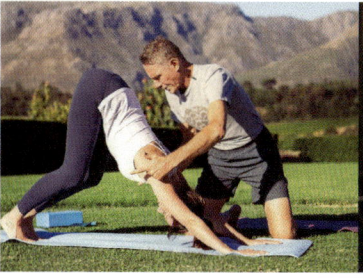
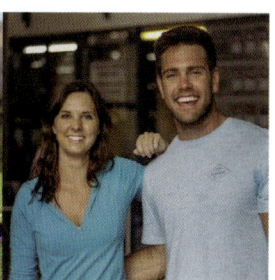

ACKNOWLEDGMENTS

The BODY BEFORE SKILL™ journey is one that has involved several experts, esteemed colleagues and dear friends. They have been my teachers, source of inspiration, challengers, supporters but most of all, my constant drive to keep feeding my curiosity.

The last 15 years, I have had the privilege to be taught by some incredible trainers from a wide variety of physical disciplines. I want to pay special thanks to my dear friends and colleagues during my two years in Stellenbosch, South Africa, where the BODY BEFORE SKILL™ method materialised into existence, as a result of extensive research, experiments and these collaborations.

I have pushed myself beyond my wildest expectations, have learned so many new concepts and explored entire new fields of movement. I have fixed my body to build stronger foundations for skill development and found a fresh jolt of liveliness and awareness.

I am privileged from learning from you all and thrilled to have incorporated all this knowledge into the BODY BEFORE SKILL™ Training Method.

GUIDE CONTRIBUTORS:

Lawrence Batchelor - *Technical Editor*
Henk Oets - *Photography*
Juliano Grimaldi - *Photography*
Holly Cammell - *Editor, Biokinetics*
Justin Schneider - *Editor, Movement Science*

BBS ONLINE STUDIO

Juliano Grimaldi - *Videography*
Martin Wan - *Videography*
Power Music Cheer - *Music Provider*

OUR FITNESS MODELS: *Holly Cammell, Jenay Mc Ewen, Megan Hendrickse, Jenna Pretorius*

WITH SPECIAL THANKS TO:
Vayden Beyleveld, Bernette Beyers, Maties Cheerleaders 2017, Debbie Love & the brilliant team of BBS Pilots.

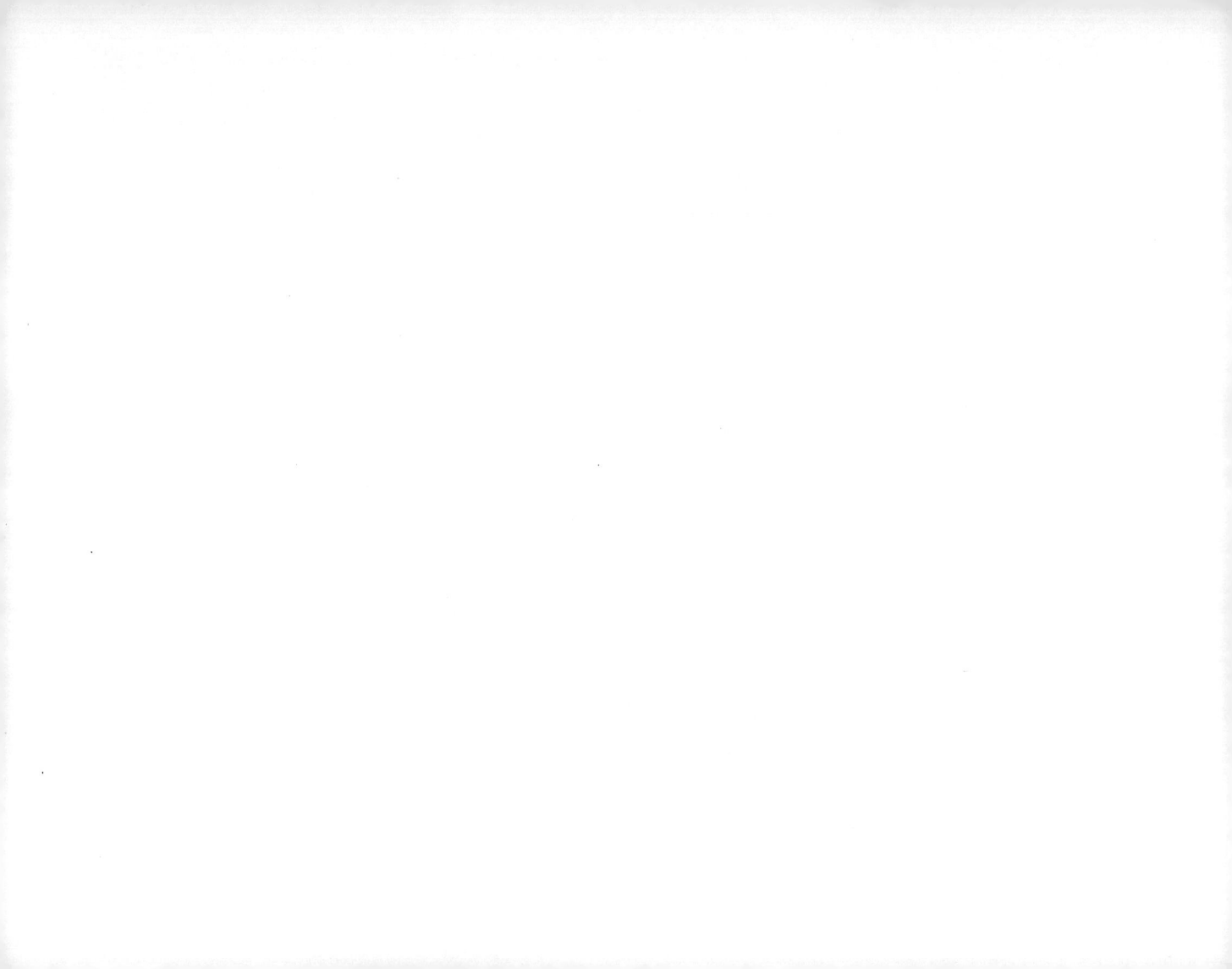

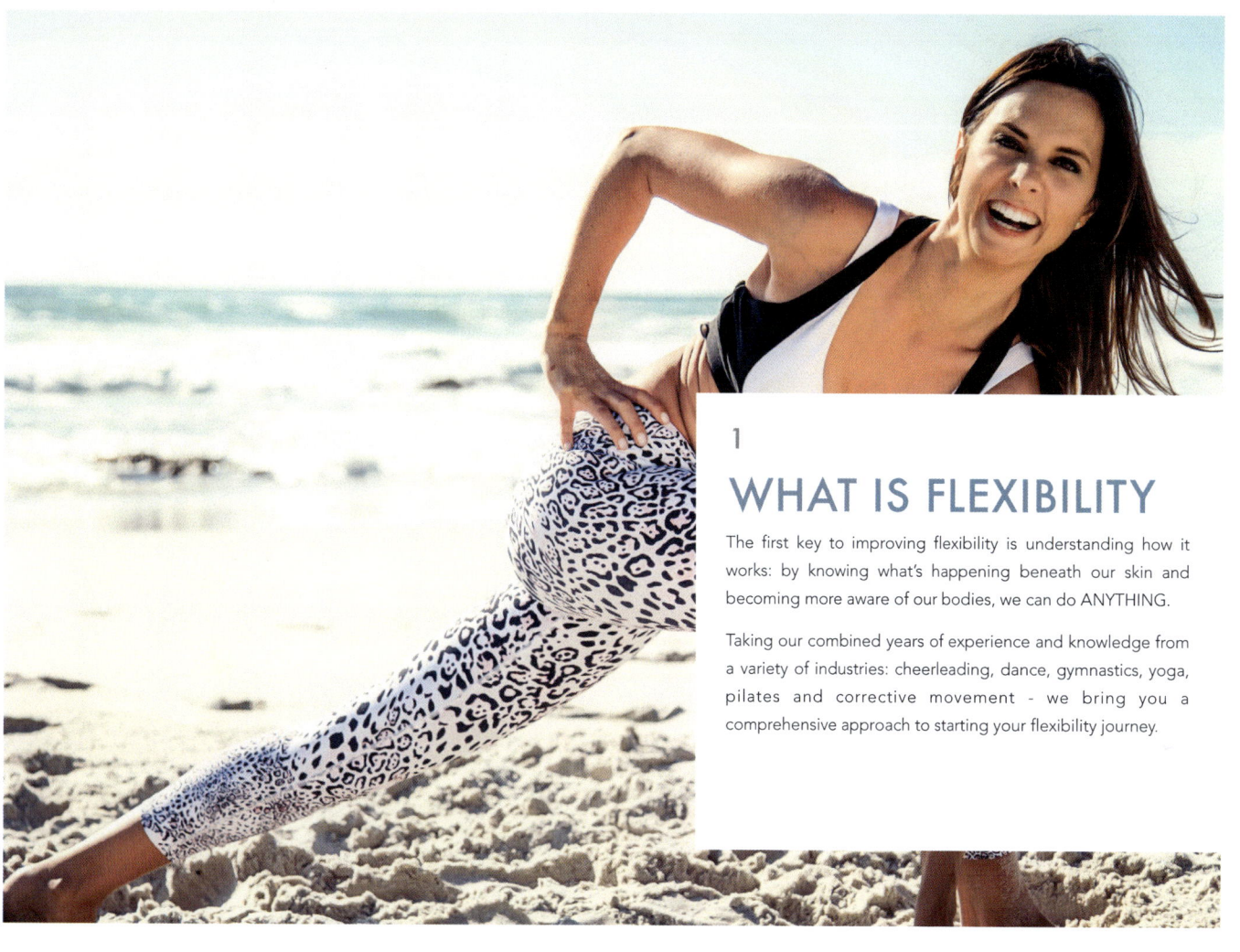

1
WHAT IS FLEXIBILITY

The first key to improving flexibility is understanding how it works: by knowing what's happening beneath our skin and becoming more aware of our bodies, we can do ANYTHING.

Taking our combined years of experience and knowledge from a variety of industries: cheerleading, dance, gymnastics, yoga, pilates and corrective movement - we bring you a comprehensive approach to starting your flexibility journey.

UNDERSTANDING FLEXIBILITY

Flexibility is *the ability of our joints and muscles to move through their full potential range of motion before reaching a breaking point.* It helps the body move more effectively and improves posture, alignment and physical appearance. It's essential to find the balance between being flexible and strong, to prevent stretching from becoming dangerous.

When we speak of flexibility, the most important thing is to recognize the difference between:

RANGE OF MOTION: the distance and direction the joint can move: it's the measurement of the movement around a specific joint, taking into account the mechanics of the joint. *E.g. Maximum movement when trying to touch your toes.*

EXTENSIBILITY: the ability for the muscles or joints system to stretch in length: without considering control or strength. *E.g. How far your muscles and joints will stretch when trying to touch your toes.*

ELASTICITY: ability to return to its original length after stretching. *E.g. the ability of your muscles and fibres to go back to normal after a long stretch.*

STABILITY: ability to stay in control and alignment during a stretch. Good stability/control can prevent injuries from happening. *E.g. your ability to hold a heel stretch with your hips squared and correct posture.*

MOBILITY: the ability to move multi-directionally through a range of motion, taking into account flexibility and stability together. *E.g. How far you can touch your toes, safely and in full control if someone is pushing your stretch.*

ECCENTRIC STRENGTH: The ability to apply strength to your flexibility. It's the result of being able to co-ordinate actions of muscles, tendons, and neuromuscular system in an extended position. *E.g. How high can you hold your leg up without using your hand, the wall or a strap?*

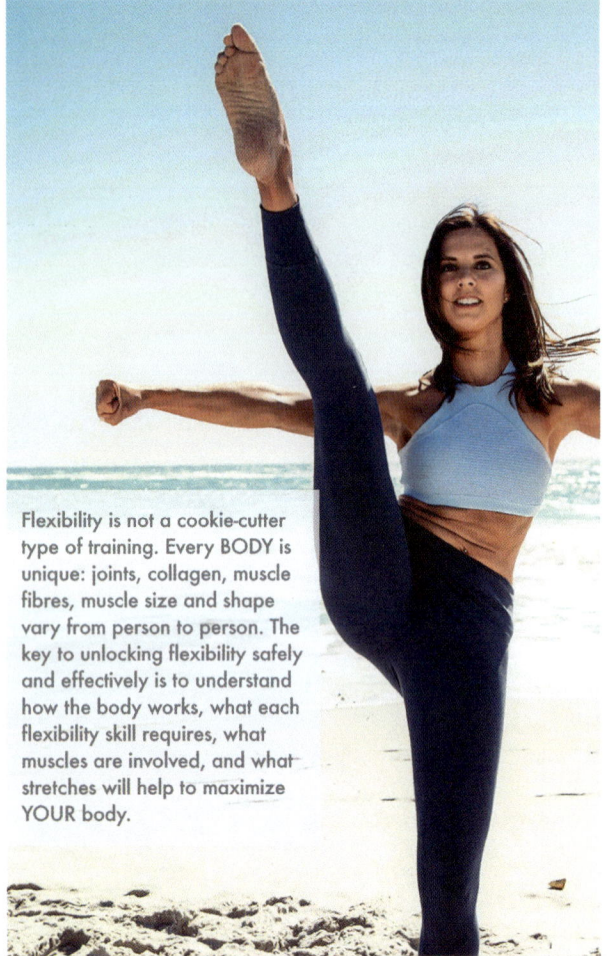

Flexibility is not a cookie-cutter type of training. Every BODY is unique: joints, collagen, muscle fibres, muscle size and shape vary from person to person. The key to unlocking flexibility safely and effectively is to understand how the body works, what each flexibility skill requires, what muscles are involved, and what stretches will help to maximize YOUR body.

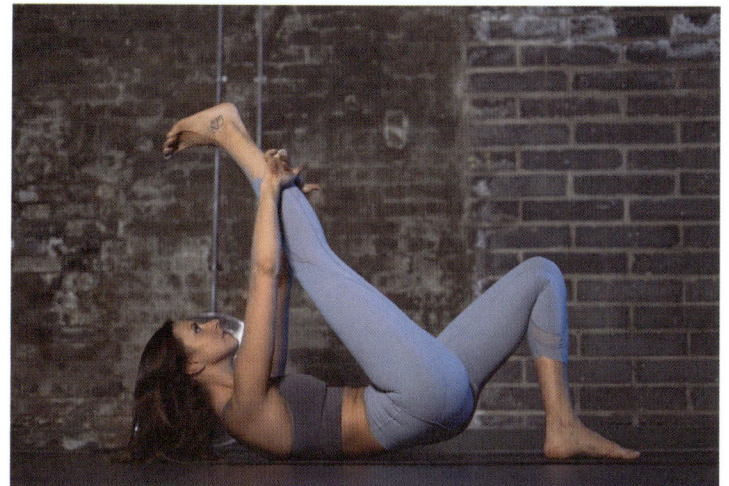

PASSIVE FLEXIBILITY

Passive flexibility relies on an external force to bring your stretch to its full range.

This means you could be using your hands, a strap, a belt, momentum, or another person. This type of stretching increases the extensibility of your fibres and your passive range of motion. It brings you to maximum stretch and your body to become more flexible, and you should relax - *not squeeze - in a passive stretch exercise.*

Use as part of your flexibility training to restore muscles after a workout or to increase your flexibility.

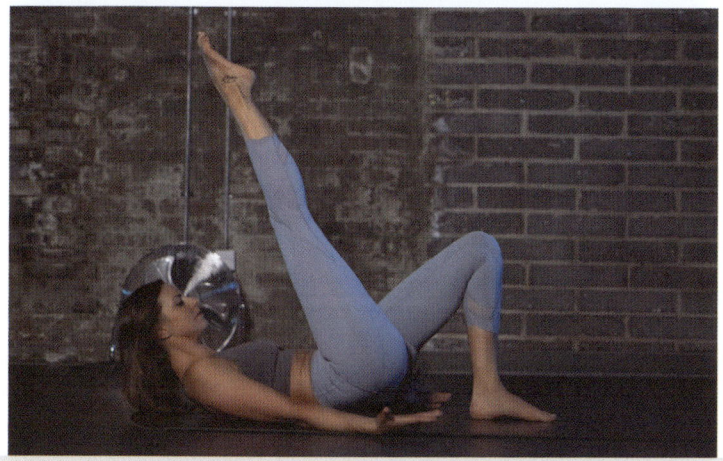

ACTIVE FLEXIBILITY

Active flexibility relies on your body's ability to reach your maximum range without an external force.

This type of stretching requires your body to dynamically move into and hold your stretch. It helps to reinforce the flexibility by adding muscle contractions and relying on joint stability.

Active stretching is very similar to eccentric and isometric strength: you're working on strengthening while the joint extends into position. This is key to maintain and develop long-term flexibility. Your active range will be smaller.

Use as part of your flexibility to develop skill and stability.

DIFFERENT TYPES OF STRETCHING

STATIC: Holding a stretch position with little or no movement. Static holds are the safest way of developing flexibility as long as muscles are warm and combined with the recommended breathing technique in Section 2, for maximum results. Learning the correct hold for each stretch statically first is crucial before you start adding movement and the more advanced stretching techniques below. Avoid static stretching during warm up to avoid weakening your muscle fibres and joints, which can reduce explosiveness and stability during your training.

DYNAMIC: Once you are familiar with the technique for a static stretch, use controlled movement patterns to increase your range. Dynamic stretches will increase the range of motion, and you can develop more flexibility by adding 3-dimensional movement. It helps to keep the muscles warm and active. It's essential to control the action so that the stretches do not become ballistic. To avoid this, keep muscles engaged and controlled. Stay in charge of the movements, squeeze in and out of your range instead of swinging or bouncing. You can use dynamic stretching after your warm up to prepare the body through mobility, without losing explosive power and stability..

BALLISTIC: This happens when you're no longer in control of a stretch, and you're submitting to an external force to push your range (such as a strong momentum or gravity). You will see this when athletes "bounce" their stretches. This technique could be risky: avoid this, especially during warm up. Fewer and fewer coaches in all sports are using ballistic stretching because of how dangerous it can be, especially when other forms of stretching can be even more useful. Our recommendation: stay away from ballistic stretching unless you are supervised by a highly experienced coach or you have suitable experience in this technique.

PNF: (Proprioceptive Neuromuscular Facilitation) This style of stretching works against a controlled force (with a partner, barre, exercise band, prop). It's useful for long-term flexibility and is also great for partner work. Again, it should not be used as a warm up before a practice or strength training so that you don't lose power and stability.

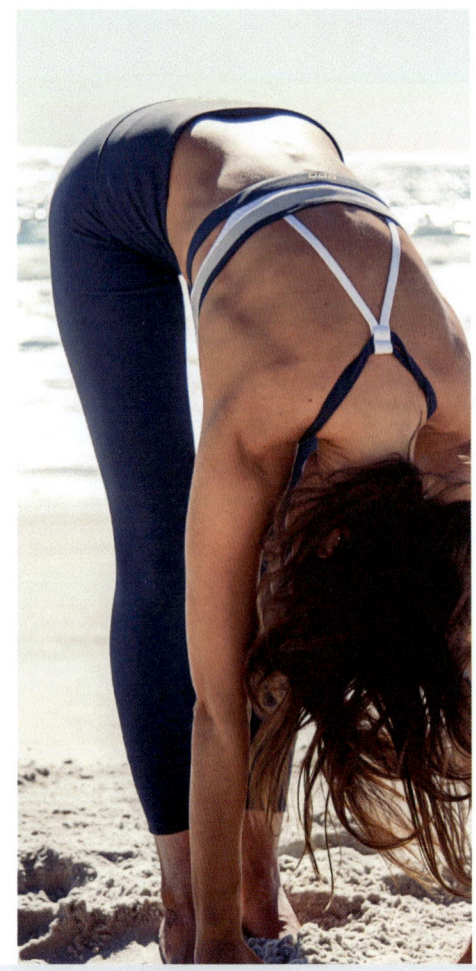

WHEN TO STRETCH

To fully understand how stretching works, we need to delve deeper than just the concept of 'warming up' before training. The balance and timings are delicate, common misconceptions of this exact science are what causes a large number of injuries in many sports.

BEFORE TRAINING: Stretching before training should only be preparatory, never developmental, as this will cause joints to become less stable and weaken muscle fibres, causing potential sprains, strains or dislocations. Preparatory stretches include dynamic movements (e.g. high kicks, side lunges), or basic held stretches. The key is to reach your current range of motion, not to push it further.

Dynamic stretching is an ideal warm up stretch. It uses controlled movement to get to your maximum range of motion available on that day, without pushing further. The movement also helps to keep the muscles warm. It's essential to maintain control so that the stretches do not turn into ballistic stretching.

AFTER TRAINING: Flexibility training (or developmental stretching) focuses on increasing the long-term flexibility and help to reduce DOMS (Delayed Onset Muscle Soreness). Spending 5-10min at the end of a training session is a necessity to prevent injury and ensure we keep developing our flexibility. Developmental stretching should also be done at home or in a separate class if you want to improve and build your flexibility further.

Flexibility is a result of genetic and training combined: one needs to make up for the other. To see an improvement in flexibility, you will need to stretch daily, using specific techniques. Once you've reached your desired range, then you can train 2-3 times a week to keep your gains.

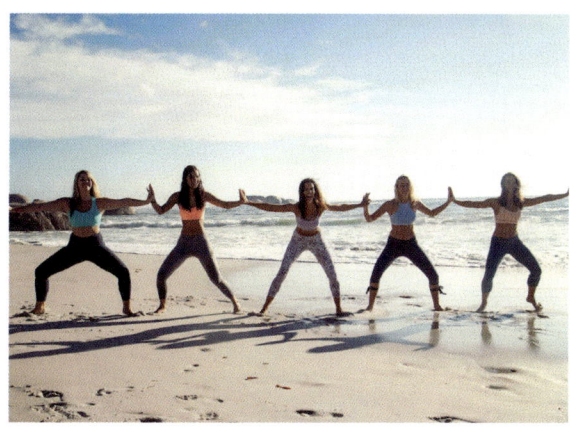

BEFORE YOU STRETCH: WARM UP.
The muscles should always be warm. Your body needs a solid 5-10min warm up to help all joints and muscles reach a higher stretching tolerance. Warm up before starting any flexibility work: whether it's preparatory or developmental.

Breathing deeply and slowly, as well as being in a relaxed environment will have a HUGE impact on your progress: your nervous system needs to be calm to increase your range. If you try to stretch when you're rushed or feeling under pressure or stress: your nervous system will stop your body from progressing further because it's stuck in "fight or flight" mode. z

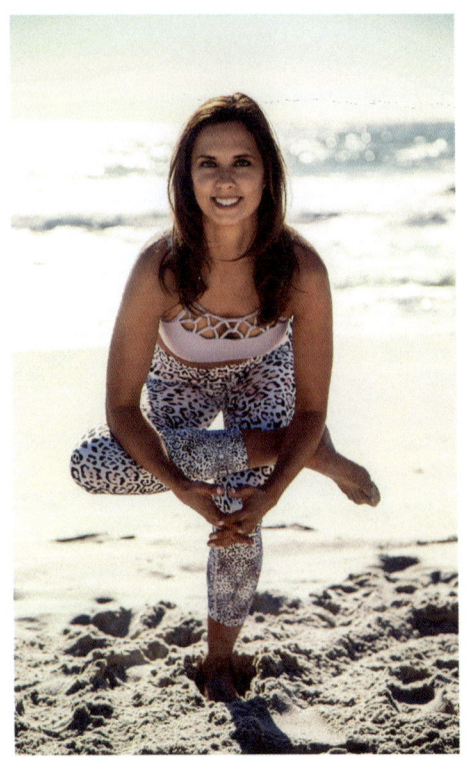

WHAT HAPPENS TO YOU WHEN YOU STRETCH?

Understanding what's happening inside our bodies is vital to help us improve flexibility. If you know how a stretch works and you're visualizing the mechanics, you have better chances of developing it. This means you'll be able to see more progress quickly.

Flexibility is our body's ability to move through our maximum range of motion. It combines muscle fibres becoming more tolerant before they tear (like an elastic band) and the joints becoming more adaptable to larger movements. Many people think that the only thing stretching is our muscles. It's much more than that:

MUSCLE FIBERS: They can stretch up to 150% before tearing. They relax and stay active during the stretch to keep control of the movement. The structure (mainly collagen) around the fibres re-model and adapt to keep the length if you stretch daily.

FASCIA: The sticky tissue made of collagen that that wraps the muscle fibres. Fascia gives structure to the muscle and makes up to 30% of your muscles. It's very malleable and contributes up to 40% of your full stretch. Research shows it also plays a crucial component in movement.

LIGAMENTS: They connect bone to bone inside a capsule. They hold the joints together. They move when you stretch, but they are not flexible. Too much stretching can cause a **strain**.

TENDONS: They connect your muscles to your bones, and they hold the position of the joint. They are very stiff and have no flexibility. Too much stretching can result in a tear or a **sprain**.

SYNOVIUM: It's an oily liquid that lubricates your joints. If it's cold, it cannot work correctly: this is one of the reasons your body needs to be warm before stretching.

STRETCH REFLEX: It's not just your muscles and joints working on flexibility; it's your nervous system as well. Imagine yourself on an ice rink with slippers on your legs will start to drift apart and you will instinctively try to bring your legs together without thinking about it. This phenomenon is the stretch reflex, and it's always working against us when we stretch. The less control you have in the stretch, the more the stretch reflex will try to over-compensate. Each year you grow older, the stretch reflex becomes more tenacious, and you become stiffer. The best way to reduce the stretch reflex is teaching your body you're in control of your movements and by stretching regularly.

PREVENTING FLEXIBILITY INJURIES

CHEATING: The temptation to 'cheat' to achieve a stretch. When we find it difficult to reach the full range of motion in a stretch, it's tempting to reach further by bending limbs, twisting hips or arching our back. "Cheating" is dangerous for our posture and joints. Be honest with your current ability, stretch regularly without "scrunching", and you will get better results.

LOSING CONTROL: Don't allow dynamic stretches to turn into ballistic movements. When stretching dynamically, our bodies can sometimes lose control over those movements. Lack of control can turn into ballistic stretching. Ensure you are extending your range safely and effectively: use slow music, think carefully about breathing and stabilisation technique.

UNREALISTIC GOALS: When we see influencers or athletes pulling extreme stretches, it's easy to want to gain that level of flexibility overnight. Chasing hyper-flexibility can lead to unsafe stretching. It will compromise the stability of the joints and can lead to injuries, especially to muscles and ligaments. It can really have severe short-term and long-term effects on the body, such as damage or stunting growth. Again, we'd say: be honest with yourself, stretch regularly with correct form, warm up properly. You WILL progress healthily in your flexibility: to benefit your skills and your body.

POOR TIMING: Only train developmental flexibility after practice or a workout, never before. Stretching for flexibility before training can cause serious injury as you are weakening your muscle fibres and joints that need to be at their healthiest for the power and strength skills. Your joints and muscles will be weak even 24 hours after intensive stretching, meaning you are at your most vulnerable for injuries at this time. Try to avoid an intense flexibility session in the 24hours before a big training session or practice. Especially when you're in competition season: don't work on pushing your flexibility skills further. A heavy focus on developmental flexibility training during intensive training or competition season can cause injury. Instead, this is an excellent time to focus on stability and active stretching.

> **ALIGNMENT:** your ability to keep joints stable and balanced during movement. Stay focused on your stretch and focus on correct technique to stay in alignment. This will help you to prevent injuries during and after stretching.

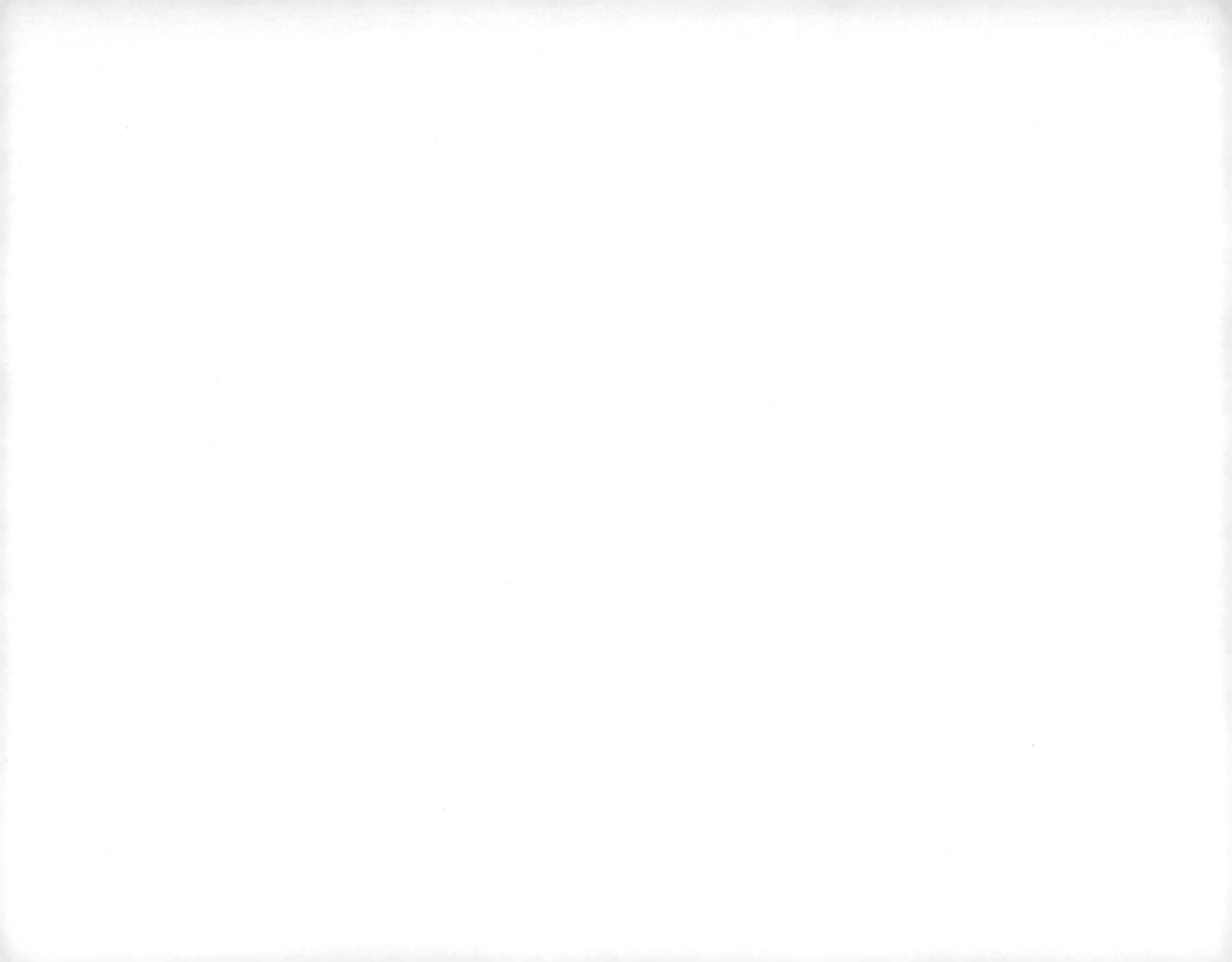

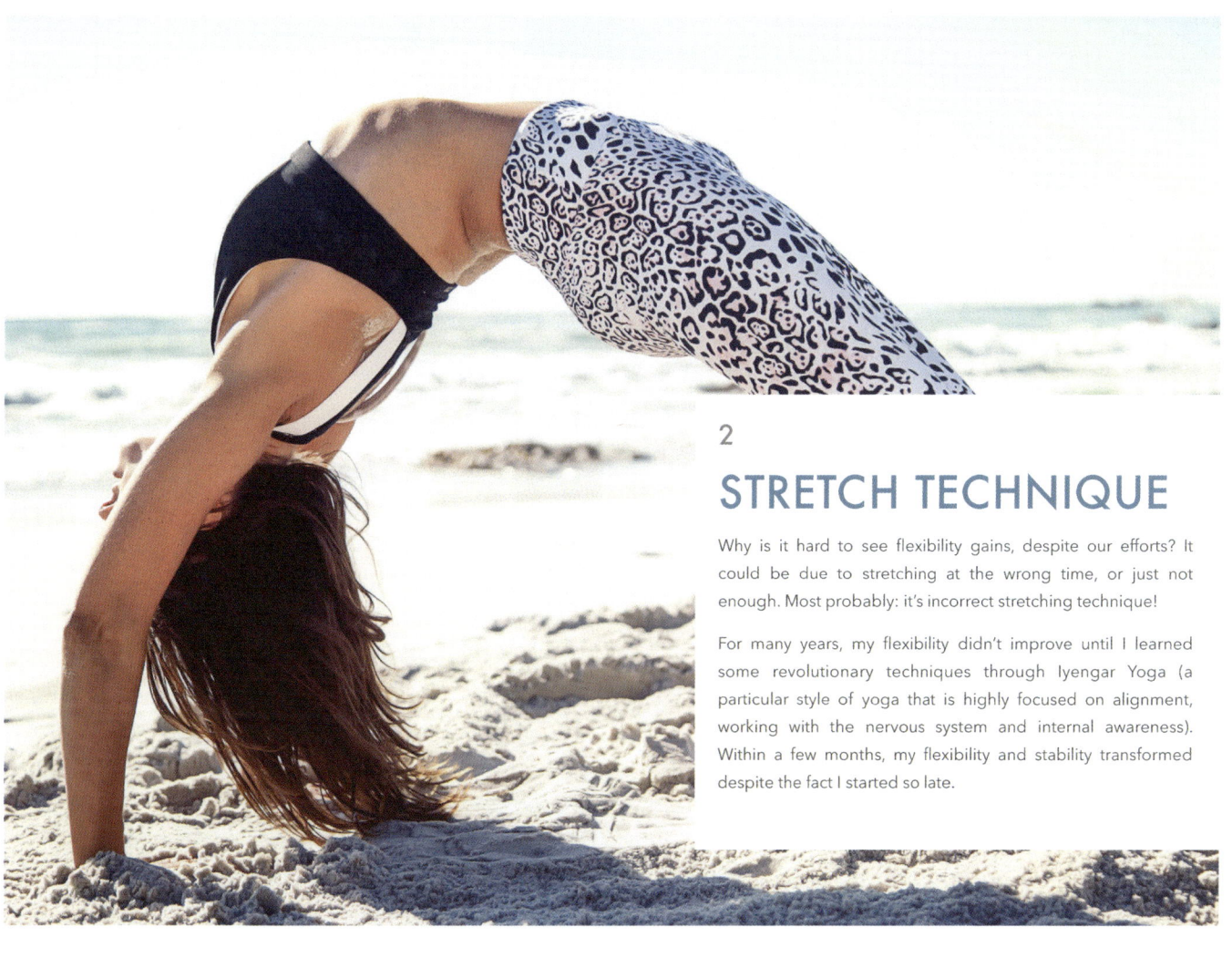

2

STRETCH TECHNIQUE

Why is it hard to see flexibility gains, despite our efforts? It could be due to stretching at the wrong time, or just not enough. Most probably: it's incorrect stretching technique!

For many years, my flexibility didn't improve until I learned some revolutionary techniques through Iyengar Yoga (a particular style of yoga that is highly focused on alignment, working with the nervous system and internal awareness). Within a few months, my flexibility and stability transformed despite the fact I started so late.

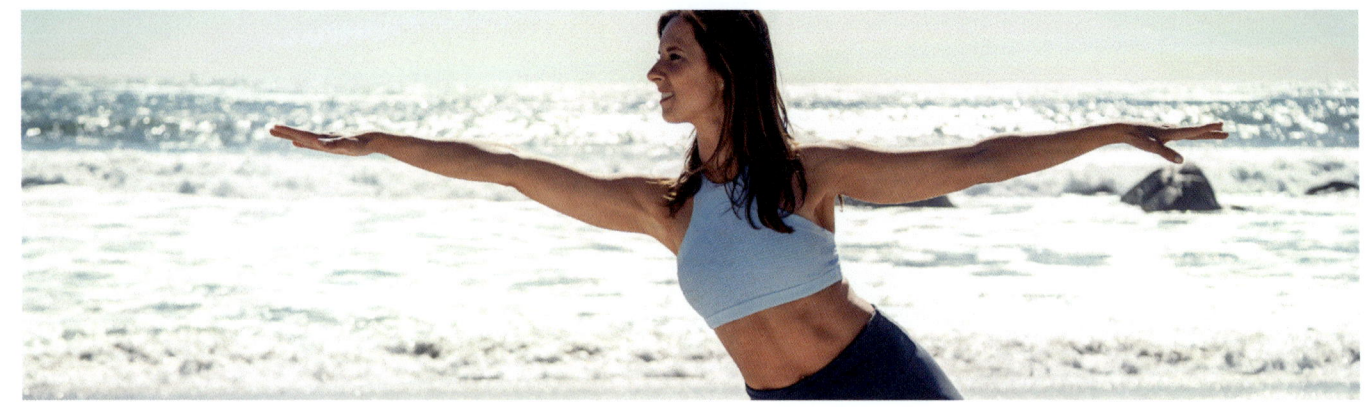

STRETCH LONG

It's tempting to feel competitive when we stretch or find a more comfortable way to reach the end range. We end up scrunching rather than lengthening into the position. This is our body "adapting", but it often translates into misalignment and poor technique.

It's our subconscious way of coping to avoid discomfort, to make it easier. Except that it has the opposite effect on our goal, which is to lengthen the muscle fibres.

Next time you find yourself in a challenging stretch, notice if you are bending, twisting or arching to increase the range. Stop, reset, realign and remind yourself to REACH LONG into the stretch. If you're in discomfort, it means you're working the right way! Just breathe and be patient: you will soon start to see improvement. Even though right now it might look like you're taking a step back, you're not: the important thing is to feel the stretch while lengthening: not looking crooked...

STOP SCRUNCHING: it's limiting your flexibility progress! Rounding your back is ok but only in very specific circumstances (for example if you are actively trying stretch the lower or upper back).

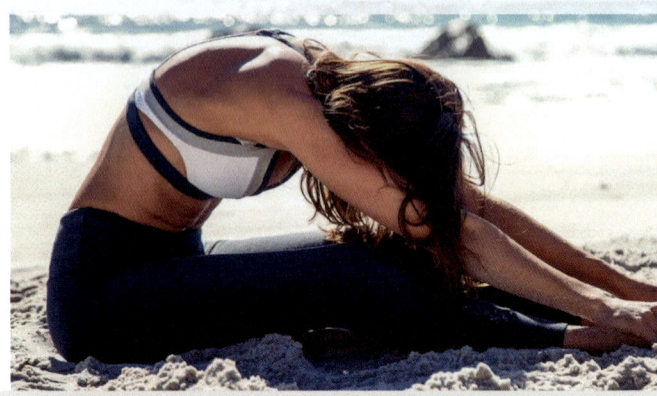

360 MOBILITY

Your flexibility training should use a combination of multi-directional movement, i.e. stretching in ALL directions rather than just pulling the skills (e.g. scorpion, splits or bow and arrow). To achieve enough of a range, you can't just be stretching one position in one direction. Each flexibility skill requires dozens of smaller muscles, and connective tissues work altogether in synergy. Using dynamic movement and 3-dimensional mobility to train for maximum flexibility is the key to skill development. Bonus: it will also help you to prevent injuries.

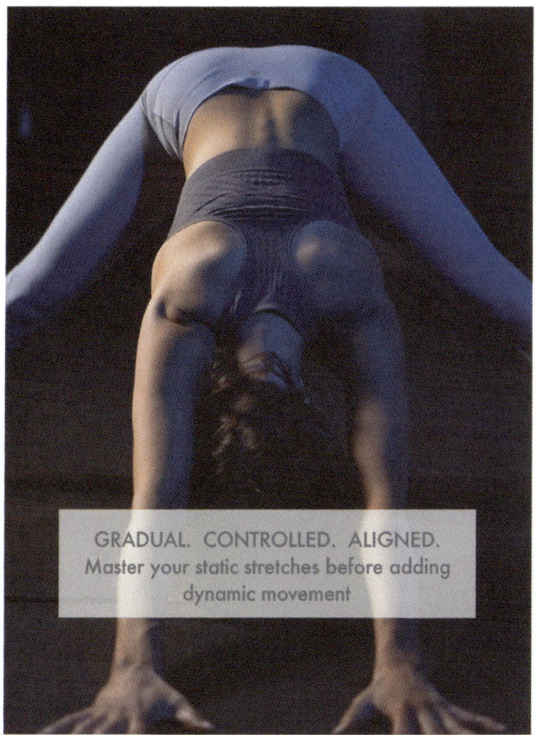

GRADUAL. CONTROLLED. ALIGNED.
Master your static stretches before adding dynamic movement

ONE GEAR AT A TIME

It's possible to notice quick progress in your flexibility after just one session. Flexibility isn't just muscles and joints: it also involves your nervous system and natural body defenses trying to protect you. If you work "with" (not against) your body and give it support during your flexibility, you will be easing the nervous system into co-operating with you instead of working against you. Calm, gradual stretching signals your nervous system that you're not in danger, allowing your defences to subside and trust your movement into a greater range.

Rather than trying to jam yourself in half in one go, aim to get into your full stretch in 3 or 4 "gears". Breathe into the stretch in gradual phases before reaching your maximum. Almost like taking a car from zero to top speed, using gears. You'll be surprised how much further you can go by using this **breathing & extending technique:**

- Get into your stretch, comfortably, with proper alignment
- Breathe in deeply
- Exhale slowly, ease further with correct alignment
- Stay in the stretch for 10-15 seconds
- Breathe in deeply
- Exhale slowly, ease further into the stretch
- Repeat twice more, and then fully relax into the end range

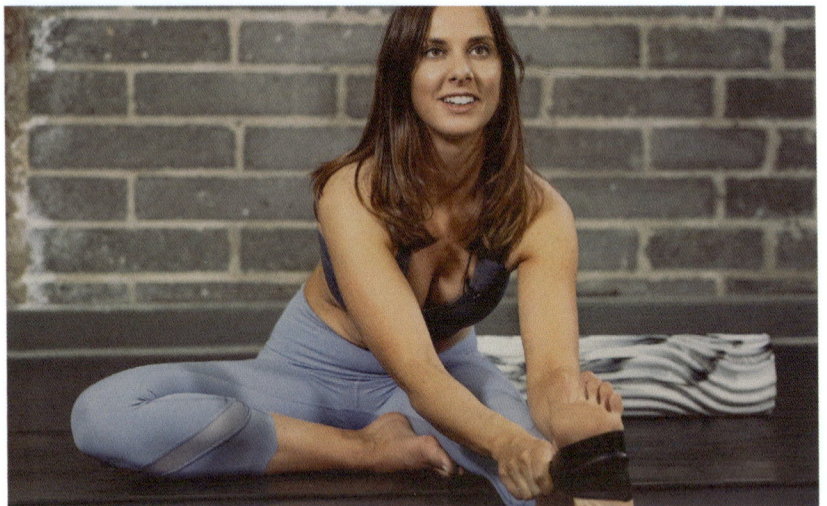

USING ACCESSORIES

If you're working on a stretch that you can't hold without compromising your technique (eg: you can't hold your ankles without curving your back) you can use some props to help. Using an accessory can make you more secured in the stretch: this means you can push further because you feel safer and more comfortable in being supported. You will also be able to work in better alignment by stretching in the correct direction.

You don't need expensive props or equipment: you can find creative ways without spending money on gimmicks or pricey tools. Some great, inexpensive stretching aids include:

- A yoga block (or a stack of books)
- A chair, stool or window-sill
- A resistance band, strap or a a belt
- A blanket
- A wall or the couch
- A foam roller
- Massage ball, peanuts or tennis ball
- Pilates or a medicine ball

CONTROL

REMEMBER: don't allow dynamic stretches to turn into ballistic movements. When stretching dynamically, our bodies can sometimes lose control over these movements.

Swinging in and out of a stretch without any control is a form of ballistic stretching, and you can quickly pull a muscle.

Always stay in control: ensure your muscles are active and you're in control of the movement.

Muscles should stay active to assist you into the stretch. Muscle activeness will depend on your stretching action:

- While you're holding a stretch passively: low/mild tension
- When you're holding a stretch actively: mild/full tension
- While you're fully relaxing into the stretch: no tension

Learn to recognise which phase/style of stretching you are using to engage muscles correctly and staying in the correct alignment. Picture the correct positions of your skill: starting, moving and into the end position.

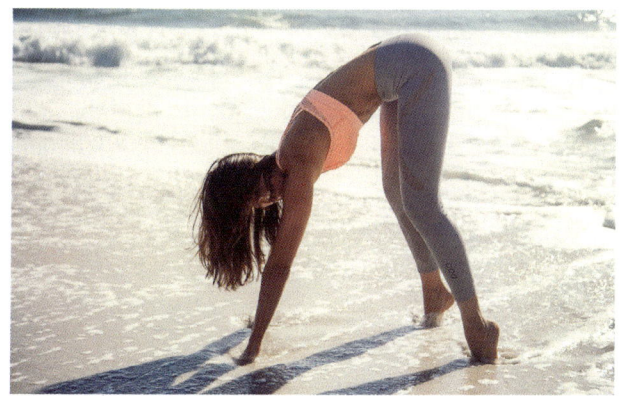

UNDERSTAND EACH STRETCH SKILL

Each stretch has a particular function and reason. It extends a different muscle group, movement chain and prepares you for a skill. The best thing you can do when you're in a stretch is to ask yourself WHY. Why are you doing this movement or position? By asking yourself this question, you can be more introspective and decide if it feels correct. If you learn to be intuitive and observe your body, you will see results more rapidly than if you're aimlessly bending, folding and copying what everyone else is doing...

SHOULD STRETCHING HURT?

Stretching should never hurt, but it can feel sore. The difference is that pain feels "sharp" and soreness feels "uncomfortable". If anything feels sharp, you should stop or reduce your stretch. If it feels uncomfortable, you might need to warm up a little more and breathe deeply into your position until it feels more comfortable. If a muscle is particularly tight, it may be a good idea to perform some myofascial release before stretching (see section 4). When you stretch properly, it's normal to feel some discomfort. Breathing deeply and easing into the stretch should increase your tolerance and make it more enjoyable.

- Have you pulled a muscle? It could be due to:
- Not warming up fully
- Excessive force on the stretch
- Little/no control of movement or force
- Poor technique/alignment
- Too much passive stretching, not enough active stretching

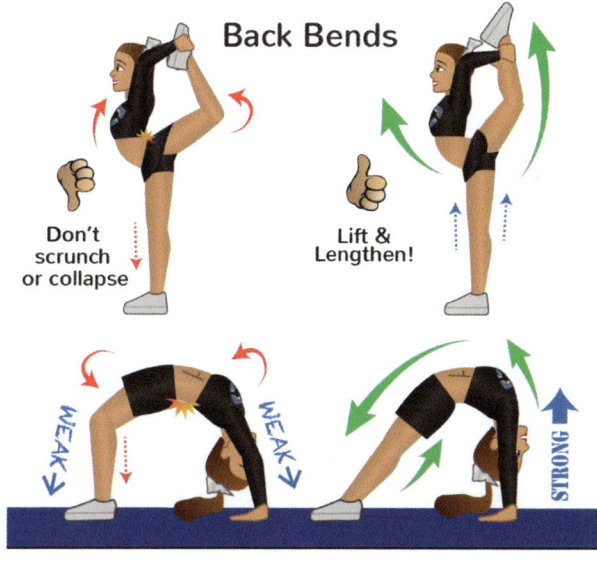

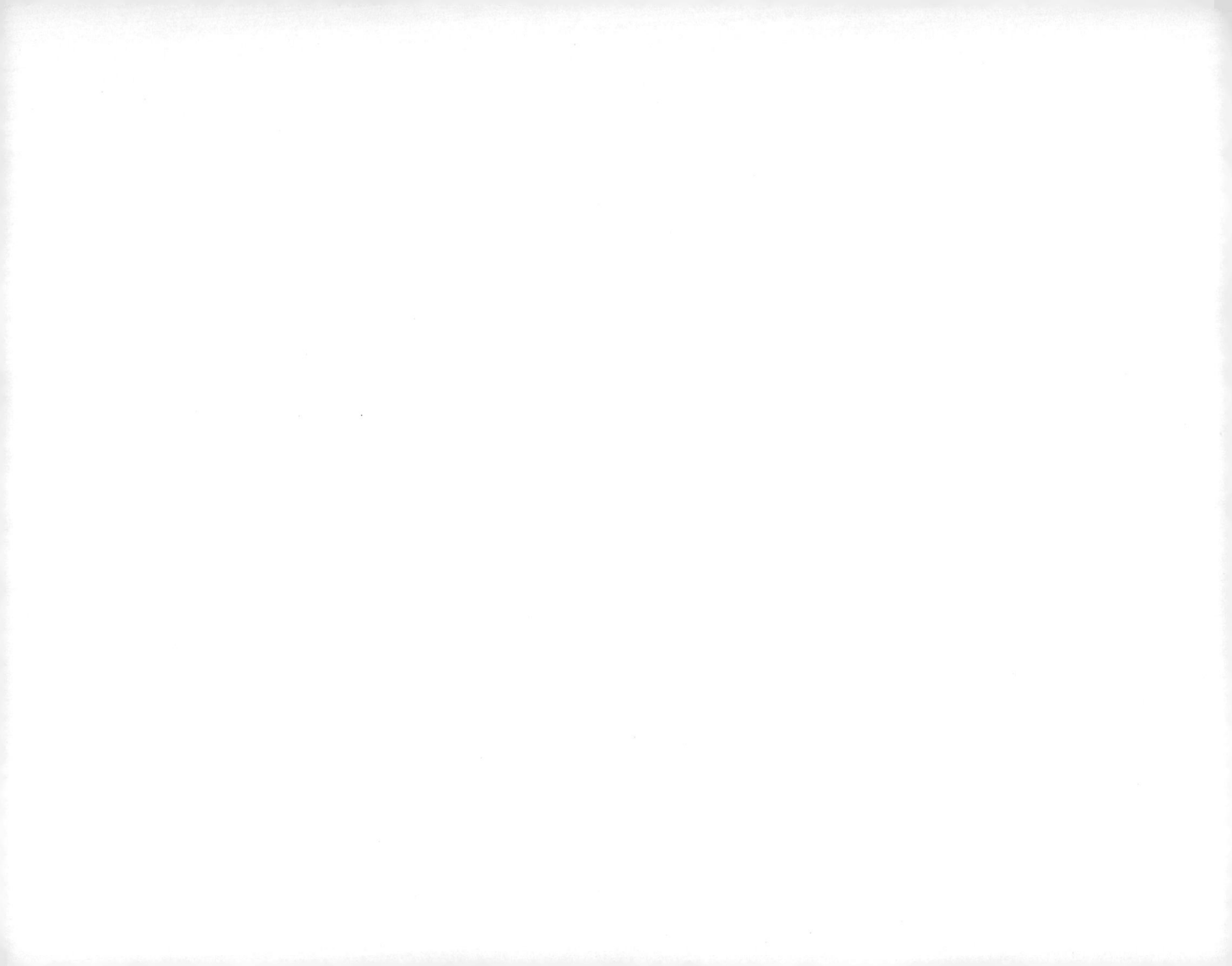

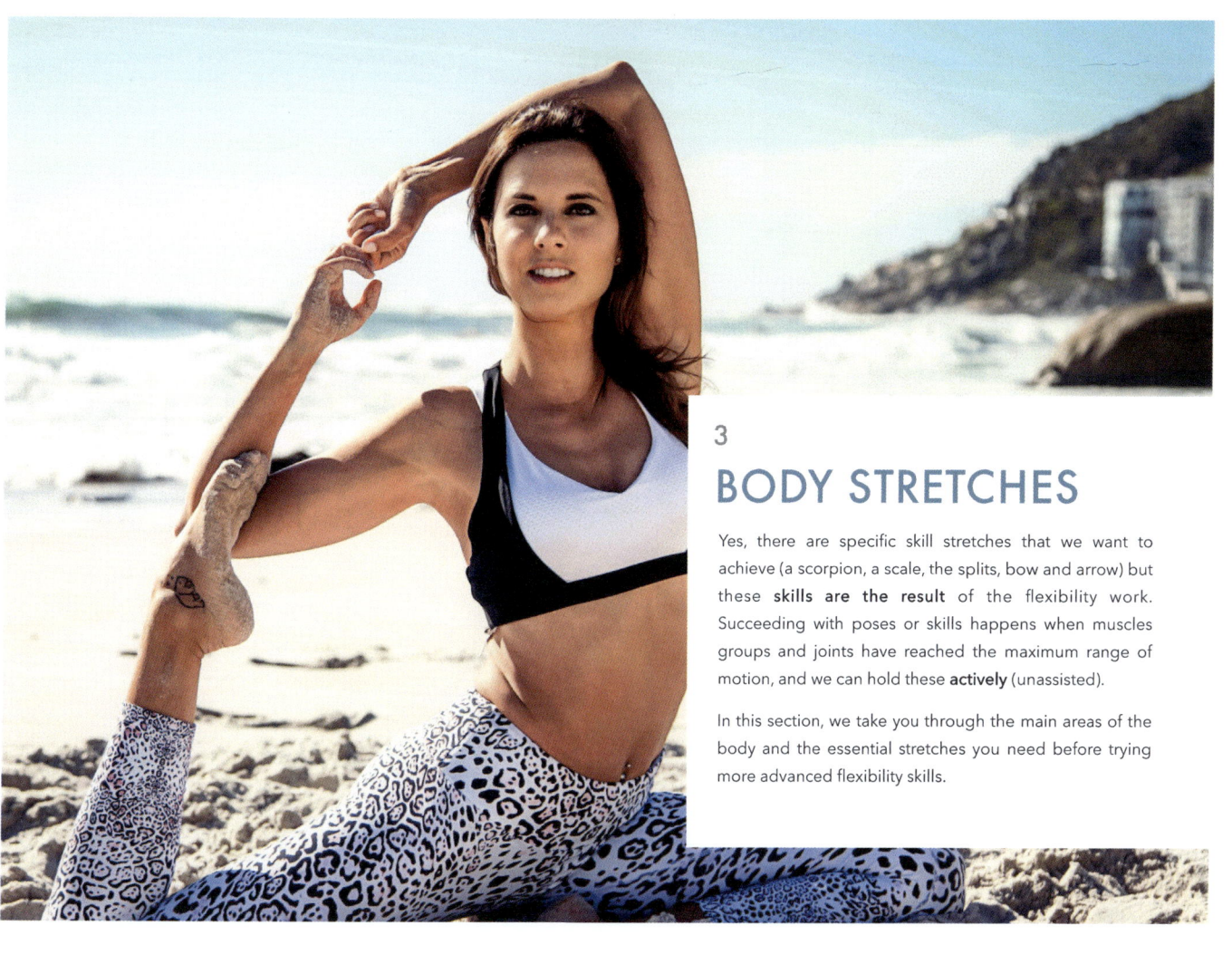

3

BODY STRETCHES

Yes, there are specific skill stretches that we want to achieve (a scorpion, a scale, the splits, bow and arrow) but these **skills are the result** of the flexibility work. Succeeding with poses or skills happens when muscles groups and joints have reached the maximum range of motion, and we can hold these **actively** (unassisted).

In this section, we take you through the main areas of the body and the essential stretches you need before trying more advanced flexibility skills.

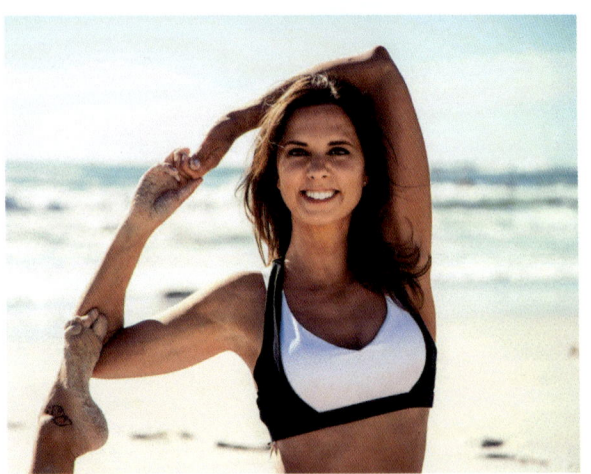

UPPER BODY

The most neglected stretch areas are the shoulders, arms and chest. This is surprising since it gets overworked more than any other muscle groups. Fitness workouts and sports tend to over-work the chest. Sitting at desks, on the couch, continually looking at our phones and driving is only making the front of our body tighter. This can result in:

- Poor posture, drooping shoulders
- Difficulty with back-bending skills
- Difficulty with overhead lifting
- Shoulder / upper back injuries

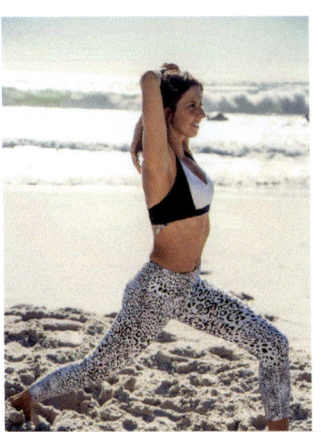

SHOULDER & TRICEP STRETCH

This is a great stretch once you're a little warm, to mobilize the shoulders, triceps and the chest. Lunge to gently stretch your glutes and quads at the same time. Keep the lower front ribs down, core strong and tuck your tailbone under to avoid arching your lower back.

Hold each side for about 15 seconds, and repeat twice.

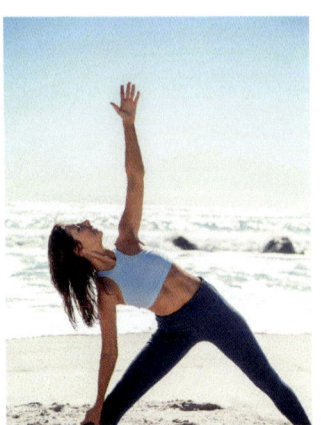

STRETCH VERTICAL

Instead of collapsing downwards when you stretch your legs, use this as an opportunity to stretch your chest.

Lengthen your spine (think long, straight and strong) and open up the opposite hand reaching up. Your hips and shoulders should be square to the front.

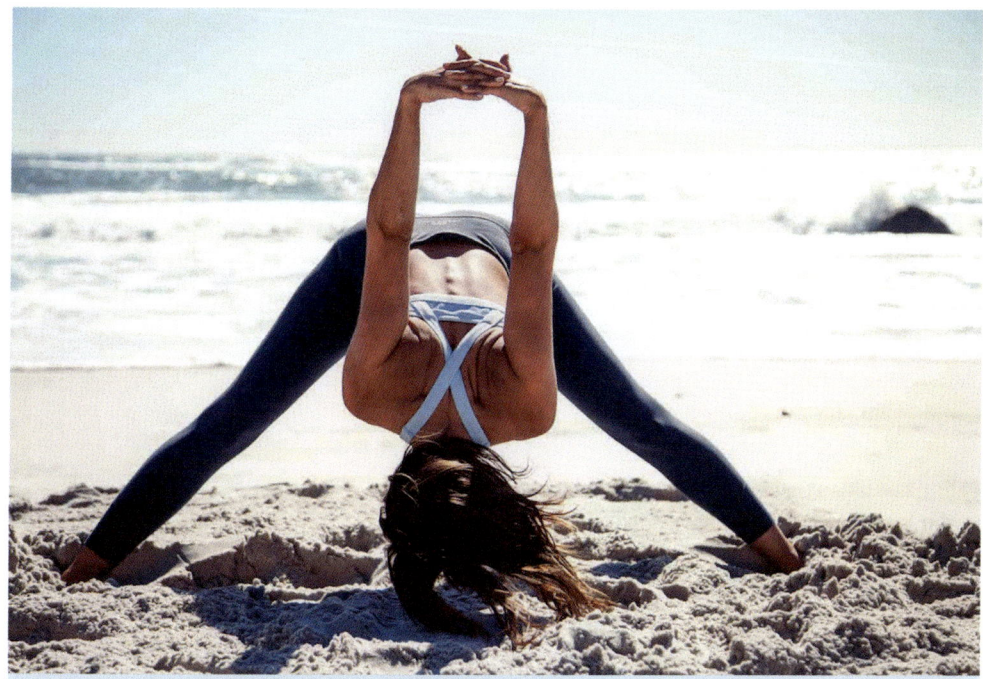

REMEMBER THE BBS BREATHING & EXTENDING TECHNIQUE:

Breathe in deeply

Exhale slowly, ease further with correct alignment

Stay in the stretch for 10-15 seconds

Breathe in deeply

Exhale slowly, ease further into the stretch

Repeat twice more, and fully relax into the end range

Get out of the stretch slowly and with control

SHOULDER CLASP

Standing feet wide apart, fold forward to bring your head to the floor. Clasp your hands behind you. Extend your back so it's straight as you reach towards the floor.

The back of the legs are long, sit bones lifting. Shoulders squeeze into the back. The front of the torso is long. Core braced. Stretch from the shoulders to the hands with arms straight.

Lengthen your arms away to the ceiling and aim to bring them to the floor in front of you. Think of unfolding long, like an accordion.

Create length in four directions:

- Between the shoulders
- Between the wrists and shoulders
- Between hips and the head
- Between the glutes and heels

GRAVITY AT WORK

If you have some extra time, it's a good idea to let gravity do some work on your shoulder and chest. It cannot be stressed enough: these muscle groups are painfully tight and over-worked. It took me six months of stretching this area to get it back to "normal". Even now I work on it weekly to keep tightness at bay.

For this method, we're letting the forces of gravity to do the work. You will need a fitness ball, a foam roller, yoga block, a pillow, sofa, chair or the side of the bed. You will need at least 5 minutes for gravity to work its magic.

NOTE: do not use weights or any external force when using gravity: this should be a gentle pull that slowly turns into comfort.

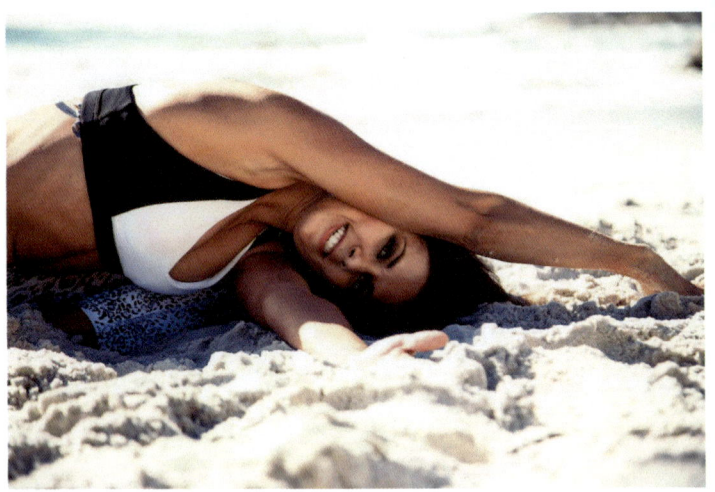

ULTIMATE GRAVITY CHEST & SHOULDER OPENER

1. Play your favorite chillout song, it will help with your nervous system.
2. Prop up your hips, back and base of the head SECURELY: make sure you're fully stable before your hands come off.
3. Engage the core and glutes: even if you're stretching the hips, this is not the time to let the booty and ribs loose or you will reduce the stretch.
4. Bring your arms straight behind your head. Shoulders down into the back of your body. Relax, breathe deeply and let the arms sink back for one minute.
5. Move your arms wider. Hold for a minute. Repeat this until you have gradually moved position with your arms wide open (see picture on the left).

When you move position, you may notice that your shoulders and chest feel tight for 20-30 seconds and the muscles adapt to the position.

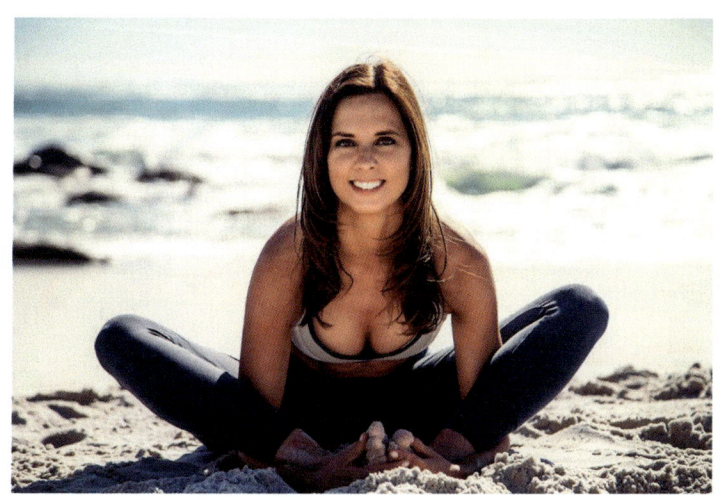

GLUTES & ABDUCTORS

Depending on if you're using your legs correctly during skills or movement in general, your glutes and abductors (side of the thighs) should be working really hard. Giving the glutes a good stretch means we need to work them at a variety of different angles. There are three main gluteal muscles; each needs to be stretched with a variety of ranges. Glutes and abductors that don't get enough stretching will result in:

- Muscle soreness and stiffness
- Difficulty to achieve splits and jumps
- Poor balance and stability
- Lower back pains

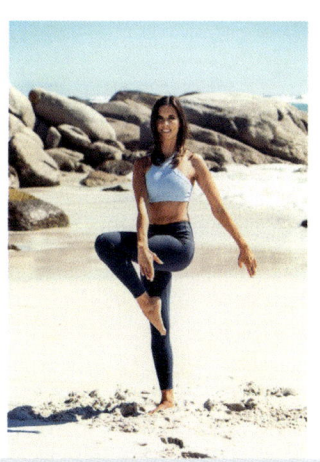

STANDING LIB TWIST

This is a great stretch once you're a little warm, to mobilise the glutes. Stand strong on one leg: knee and thigh facing forward. Lift the other leg, holding the knee at 90 degrees and foot pointing by the standing knee. Now pivot the bent leg to the back, keeping your chest forward. Rotate the torso away from the knee, lifting up, shoulders broad.

Hold for about 15 seconds, and repeat twice on each side.

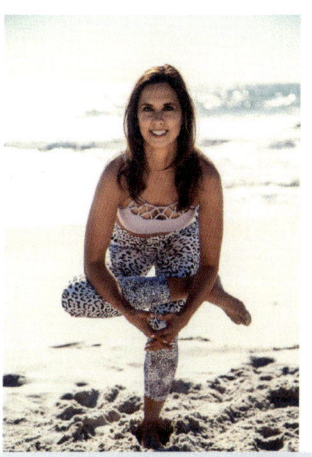

STANDING FOUR

Stand on one leg. Bend the other leg, resting the foot just above the standing knee, on the thigh. Keep hips level and sit back with control. Keep shoulders broad while you fold forward at the hips to rest your forearms on your leg. Keep the shinbone horizontal to the floor. To get a deeper stretch, bring the hands to the ground.

Hold each side for about 15 seconds, and repeat twice.

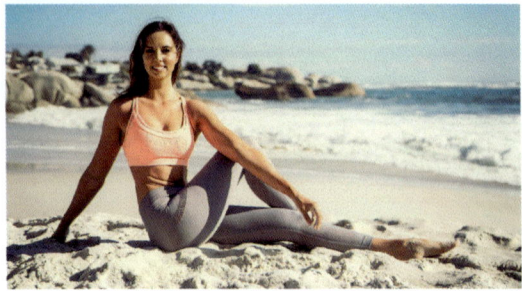

SITTING TWIST

Sit tall, facing your feet. Bend one leg and place the foot over the straight leg, outside the knee. Keep lifting tall as you pivot your torso towards the flexed hip. Squeeze the elbow into the knee, resisting with the leg. Shoulders broad, hips forward, chest lifted.

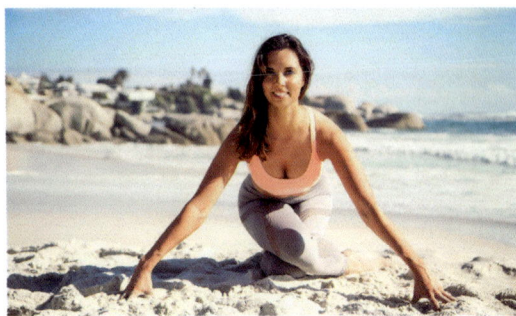

SITTING CROSS

Stand on all fours, legs together. Cross one leg over, aligning knees one behind the other. Hinge the feet out away from each other and slowly sit back between the feet. Use your hands to stay balanced. Sit on a pillow or block for support.

Hold each stretch for 20 seconds, breathing deeply into each gentle push.

Repeat on each side, twice alternating sides.

Keep hips square, spine long and chest open at all times.

If you feel your body "cheating" correct it by keeping long and straight: the stretch will be more effective.

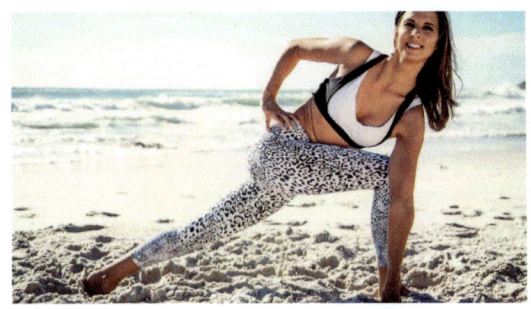

TWISTED LUNGE

Start in a deep forward lunge, with your back leg straight and forward leg at 90 degrees. Firmly plant your feet and keep hips level. Stay long, strong and straight as you twist towards your bent leg, placing your hand on the knee, shin or the ankle.

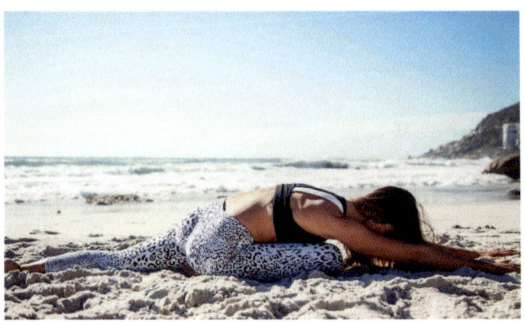

PIGEON

Kneel on all fours using your hands as support. Slide one leg back straight and follow with the hips. Bring the front foot across your chest, bringing the shinbone horizontally. Keep hips level and your back straight as you reach forward.

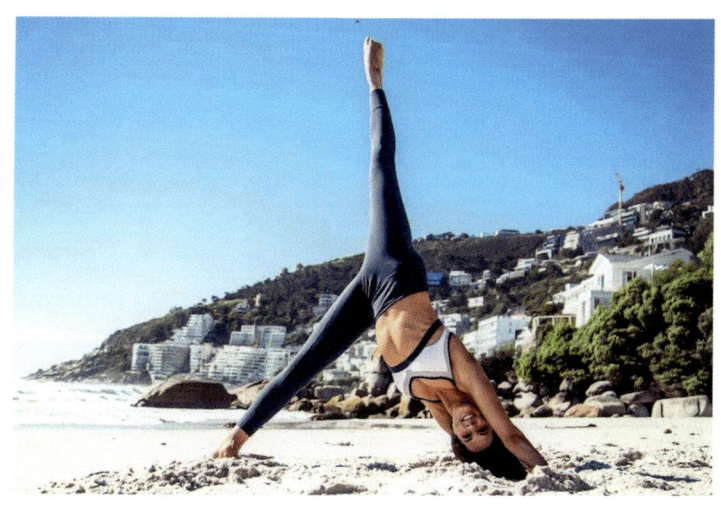

QUADS & ADDUCTORS

The quads are an intricate set of muscles at the front of the thigh. The adductors inside your legs extend between the hips and knees. Stretching this area is a crucial component of achieving overall flexibility and mobilizing the front and inside of the leg. The majority of us tend to be **Quad Dominant** i.e. using the front of the leg rather than sharing the effort with the back of the leg. This causes a variety of issues:

- Weak/inactive core leading towards lordosis
- Difficulty to achieve splits and back-bends
- Knee pain during exercise and strength skills
- Reduced leg power when quads take over: strength and stability skills are more challenging

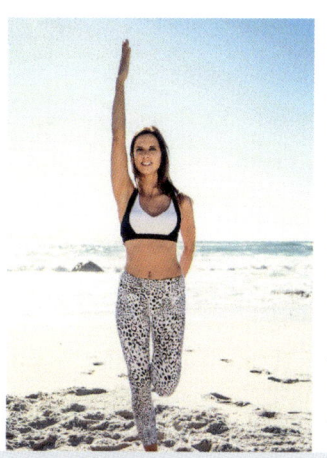

STANDING QUAD STRETCH

This is one of the most common stretches but often performed incorrectly. Holding one foot behind, squeeze knees together and push hips forward, hips fully square and level. Bring lower front ribs down but keep shoulders back: from the side you should look straight like a beanpole. Reach up with the other hand keeping core strong, spine straight and knees together. Keep the heel of the bent leg pressed against your glutes. Hold each side for 15 seconds, repeat twice.

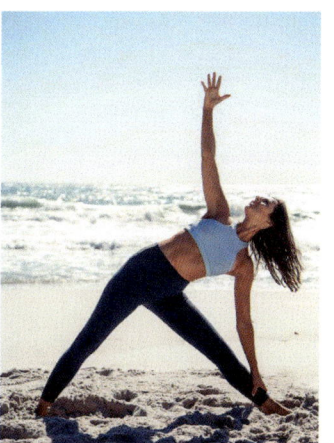

TRIANGLE POSE

Triangle pose is a really effective way to stretch your quads and adductors by adding a twisting action. The key is to stay aligned and not folding like a burrito! Start standing feet apart, tall, core strong. Reach long to one side, keeping the hips square. Pivot the torso back. Open the arms and chest to form a straight line from hand to hand. Hips forward.

Hold each side for about 15 seconds, and repeat twice.

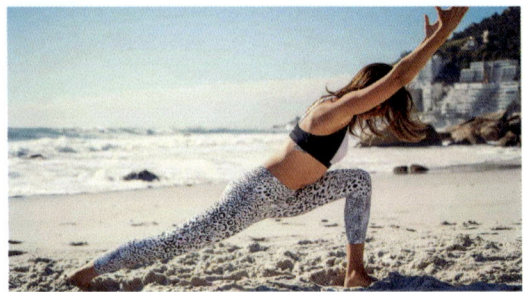

LONG LUNGE

Take a deep forward lunge with your knees strong at 90 degrees and stay lifted. Descend the hips, stretch the torso forward, lower ribs down. Feet and knees are strong, reach long, strong and straight. The back leg should be fully straight and extended.

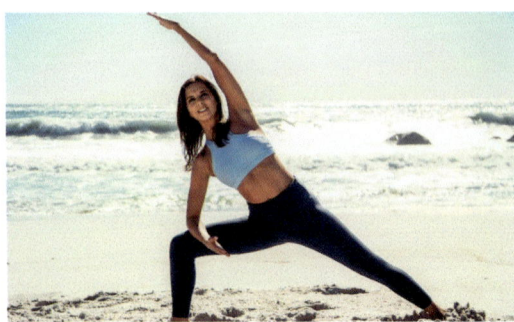

SIDE LUNGE

From your Long Lunge, move the back foot facing the front, keeping the same control on the knees and the hips. The knee faces the side, hips forward. Back leg fully straight and extended. Rest your elbow on the knee and LIFT: shoulders square.

Hold each stretch for 20 seconds, breathing deeply into each progression.

Repeat on each side, twice alternating sides.

Keep hips square, spine long and chest open at all times.

If you feel your body "cheating" correct it by staying long and straight: the stretch will be more effective.

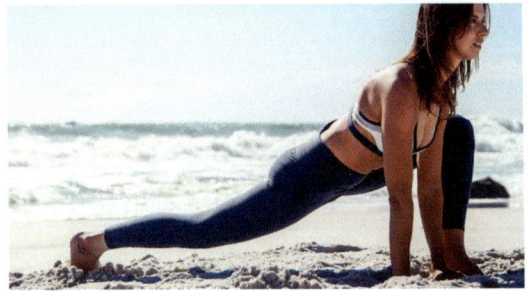

HALF LIZARD

From your Long Lunge, bring your hands inside your bent leg. The key is to keep the hips forward and lifted, chest lifted, bent knee strong (pushing away from the elbow) and the back leg straight. Imagine a straight line from your heel to your head that lengthens.

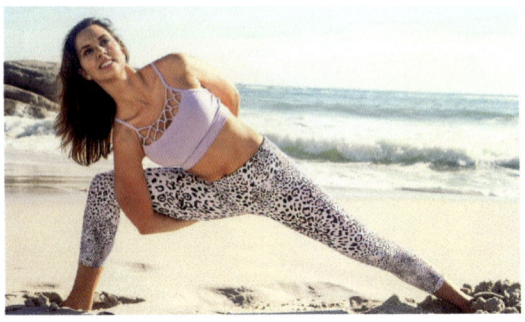

SIDE KNOT

For an extra, deeper stretch (only once you can master the side lunge correctly) slide the supporting arm under the leg, and hold the other hand. Keep lifting the hips. Back leg stays forward. Chest lifted, roll the top shoulder back, keep that long straight line.

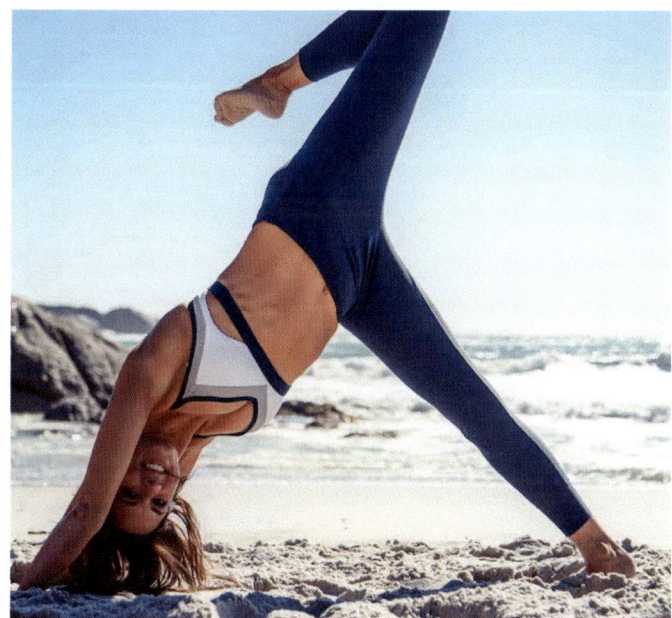

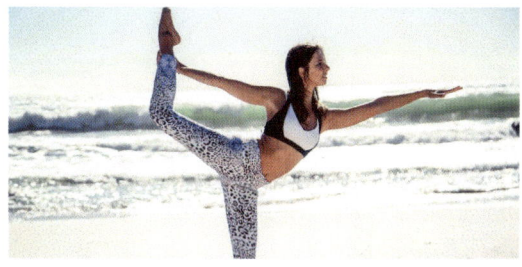

DANCER'S POSE

Dancer's pose is a CLOSED stretch. With the hips and shoulders facing forward instead of sideways, you are stretching your lower spine, hips and especially the quads. This is a great stretch to help you develop flexibility for a scale, scorpion or needle.

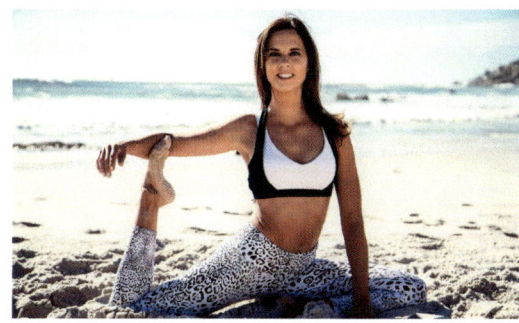

HALF MERMAID

The *full mermaid* pose (both hands holding foot at the head) is an OPEN version of a scorpion stretch (King Pigeon in yoga). If you have tight hamstrings Half Mermaid this is a great place to start. You can then attempt the CLOSED version by facing the front, with hips square and bringing your foot towards your back.

SQUARE OR OPEN HIPS?

OPEN stretches, where you open your hips to the side, are a great way to explore your range of motion. Because you're stretching more muscle groups in a 3-dimensional form, you'll notice your stretch skill becomes more open. The stretch above shows an OPEN version of the One Legged Dog which is a CLOSED hip stretch (p.29).

CLOSED stretches, when your hips remain square, and the movement is more 2-dimensional, are more difficult because they rely on an intense stretch carried out by fewer muscles. If you're trying to improve flexibility, a square position might be trying and limiting, but necessary to stretch out your tightest muscles. For every minute spent on an OPEN stretch - you should first spend two minutes on a CLOSED stretch.

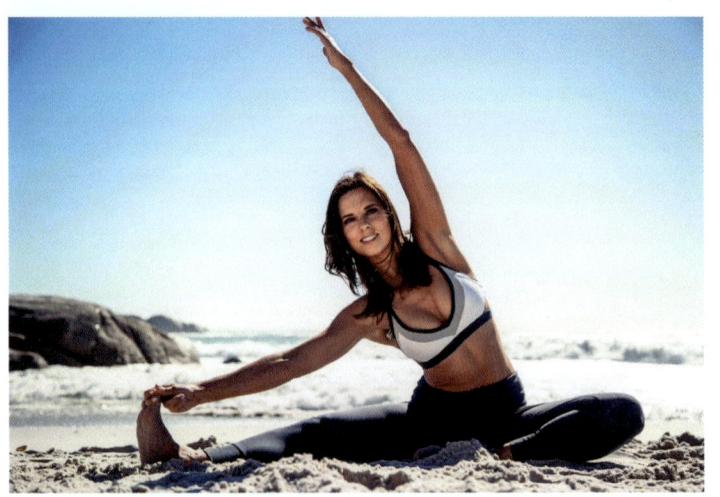

CALVES & HAMSTRINGS

The back of the legs often get very tight (even though we spend a lot of spend time stretching there). A lot of the time, instead of stretching and lengthening, we "scrunch" these stretches. This results in the pose becoming focused in our lower back rather than in the hamstring and calves. However if we focus on correct technique and alignment, we can see progress much faster. A tight posterior chain means we often see problem areas such as:

- Pulling hamstrings during stretches
- Reduced explosively and impact control
- Ankle or knee injuries when landing high impact
- Bent knees and limited flexibility in active stretch skills
- Painful calf cramps during exercise or even during rest

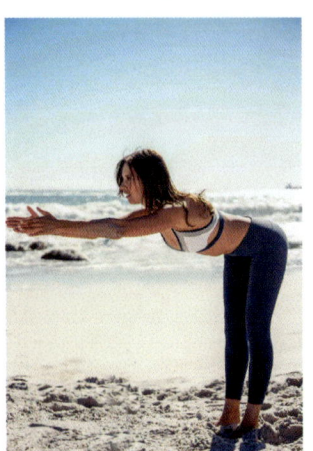

STRETCH STRAIGHT AND LONG

Learning to stretch straight and long seems simple enough, but difficult to execute without discipline and focused awareness. This was one of the biggest break-throughs that developed my flexibility. It might look like you're not as flexible when you are stretching SQUARE but you're actually targeting the muscles a lot more deeply than you would if you "scrunched" or folded like a burrito. Both these standing stretches are a great way to start warming up your hamstring and calf stretches. Notice that the spine is long: extend and straighten the line between your heels and your hips, and then your hips to the crown of your head. Hold stretches for 30 seconds.

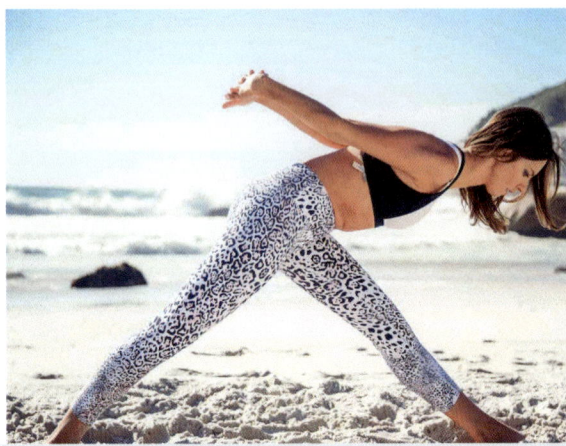

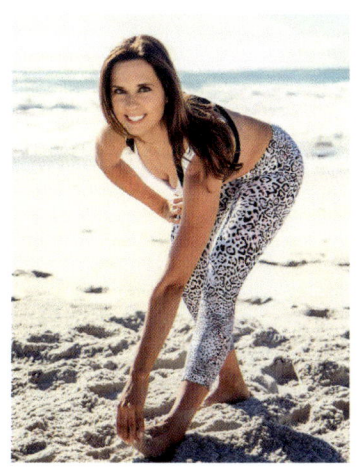

STANDING CALF STRETCH

Start by standing straight and tall, with the core strong and lower front ribs tucked in. Bring one foot forward and keep your hips square. With both hands on the hips, hinge forward keeping your back straight. Reach for the foot and flex it towards your shin. The hips, knees and shoulders should face forward while you bring your belly button to the knee. Come back up first to standing strong before you repeat with the other leg.

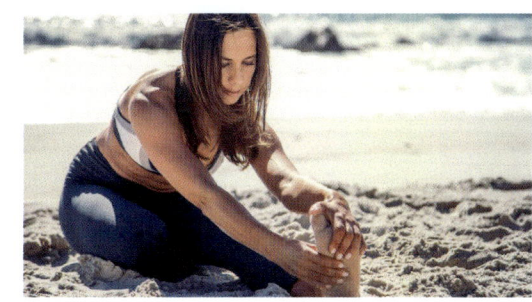

THREE PART FOLD

Sitting version of the standing calf stretch: while sitting square on your feet, extend one leg forward using the same technique. Focus on making everything square and keeping a straight line from the base of the spine to the crown of the head. Try to keep shoulders back and inside the body.

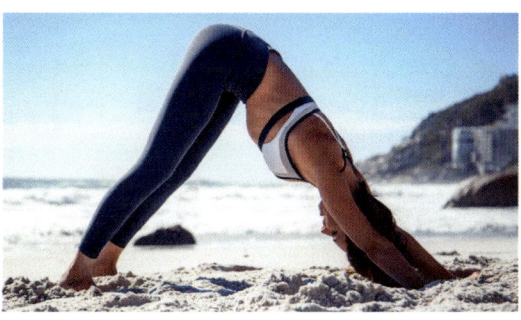

DOWN DOG

Focus on bringing your heels to the ground and your tailbone moving diagonally in a straight line away from the hands. The spine is straight and long, the core is strong and the thighs lift towards your hips. Push away from the ground by spreading and flattening the hands, reaching the heels back and down.

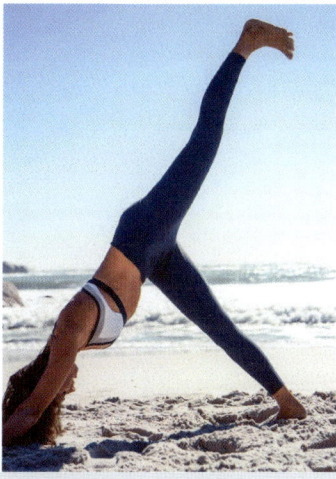

ONE LEGGED DOG

Once you feel more comfortable and aligned in your downward dog, increase the calf and hamstring stretch by extending into the heel, making one long line. The standing leg heel stretches down. This is a CLOSED hip position so make sure you're fully square with your hips, feet and shoulders: the foot is flexed towards your shin. Open your chest and shoulders, stay strong on your arms. Lower ribs back into the body.

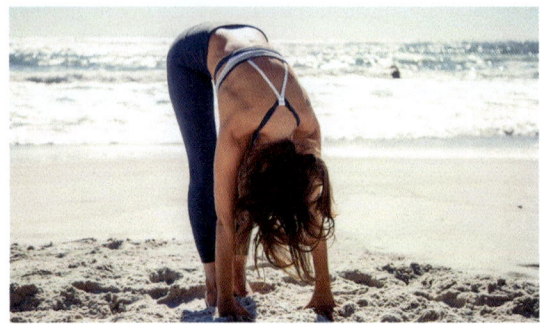

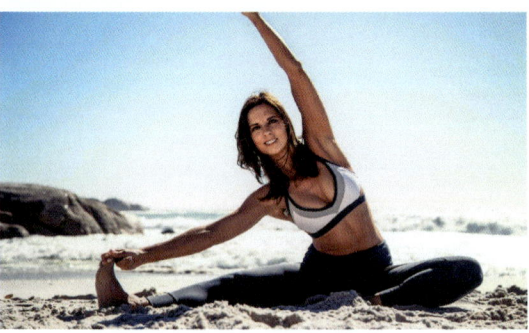

ROUND OR STRAIGHT BACK?

If you're trying to target a muscle stretch (other than your back) keeping a straight back will intensify the lengthening action of the muscles while you extend the line of stretch (see image below). Once you are comfortable in your straight stretch, you can add movement and use a rounded back to stretch other muscles, such as the lower back, and increase the visual range.

You can also round your back when you breathe in, before you straighten it again as you breathe out to deepen the stretch.

POINTED OR FLEXED FEET?

When you point your foot, the back of the leg shortens and the front of the leg lengthens. If you flex your foot towards the shins, the back of the leg lengthens and the front of the leg shortens. So if you're trying to stretch your hamstrings and calves (back of the leg), then you should stretch with your feet flexed (above).

If you want to add movement and use the stretch to work on other muscles, point you toes when you arrive at your maximum range and add another dimension of movement (below) .

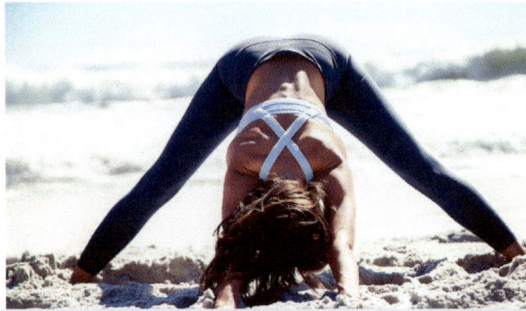

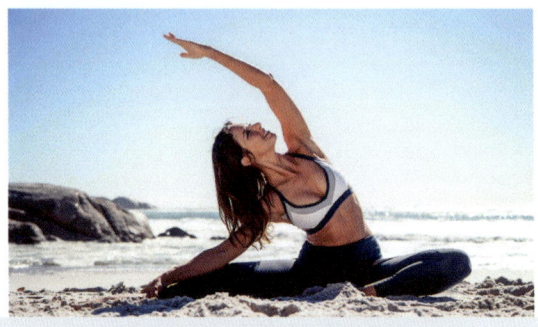

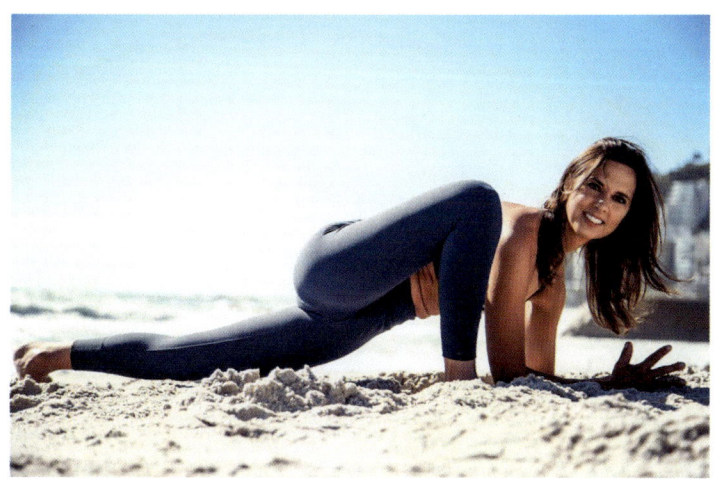

HIPS & CORE

If there is one thing that is confusing about the core and hip muscles, it is that **they can be weak in strength while also being stiff and inflexible at the same time**. The hip and the core connects our lower body to the upper body. There are many muscle groups and fibres, intricately intertwined. Hip and core mobility in this area will help you to avoid:

- Hip, adductor and lower back injuries
- Plateau in advanced flexibility skill development
- Weak core strength for acrobatics or gymnastic skills
- Calf cramps during exercise or even during rest
- Strength loss due to lower and upper body disconnection

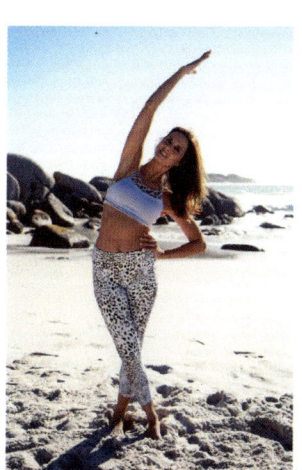

START SLOW

Before getting a deeper stretch like the Lizard (picture above) remember to start slow and mobilize the area. A simple standing side stretch (left) held for 10 seconds on each side, then repeated twice, is a great way to get going. Once you're ready you can move to deeper stretches, again in phases. To get into a full lizard stretch - get into a Half Lizard stretch with the correct alignment (right) for about 10 seconds before breathing your way deeper into the full stretch.

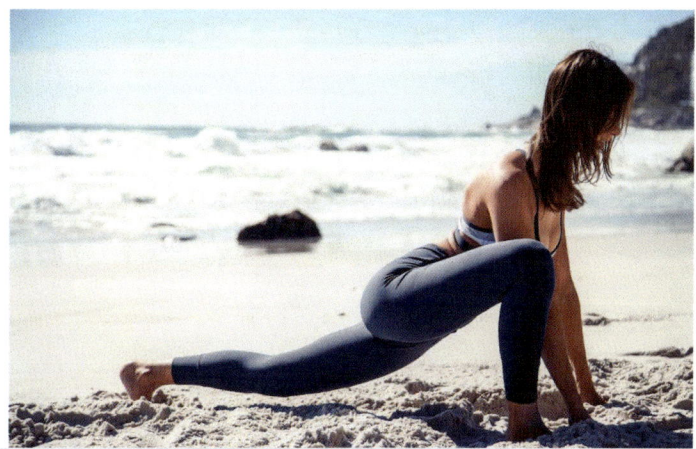

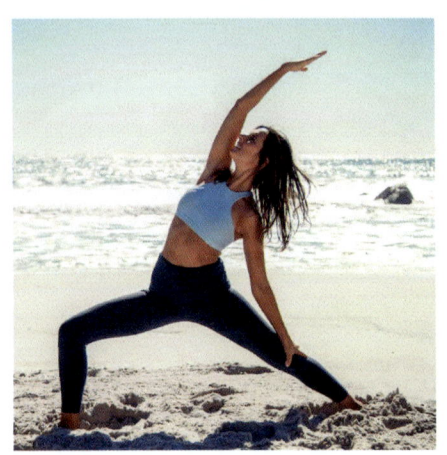

SIDE LUNGE STRETCHES

Lunge stretches (known as warrior poses in yoga) are great for opening while strengthening the hips and core muscles at the same time. Keep feet firmly planted into the ground, front knee strong and stable at 90 degrees. Front foot and knee face forward, the back foot is turned out. Torso and hips square, keeping the upper body upright. Stretch towards the back hand. Ensure you stay strong while you deepen the stretch. Hold the stretch away from the knee for 15 seconds, then pivot forward to lean into the front knee for another 15 seconds. Keep shoulders broad.

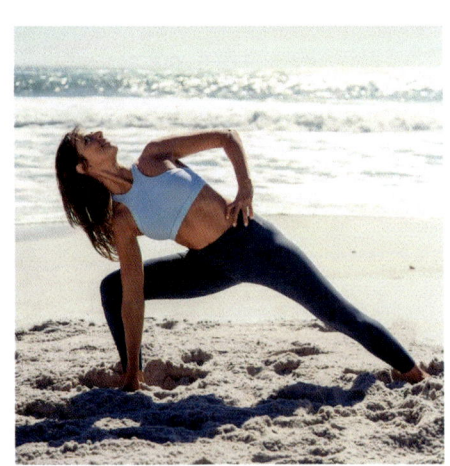

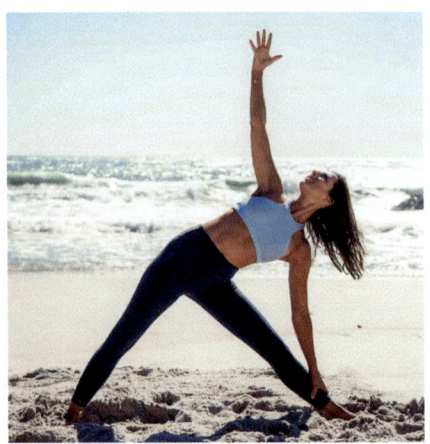

TRIANGLE POSE

The triangle pose is a great stretch that lengthens the hips, adductors and the side of the core. The key is ensuring you're forming straight lines: roll your hips and torso to face up to the ceiling, and take your torso and head back. Even though you are reaching down to open your side, the real stretch comes from pushing the hips forward and keeping your lower back neutral. Squeeze the glutes in and forward. Reach up long with your upper hand. The aim is to imagine you are making this triangle shape in a very narrow gap between two walls. Make the triangle as "thin" as you can but as tall and spread out as possible. The trick: reaching FORWARD and LONG before you pivot your torso down to the leg. Hold for 20 seconds on each side, and repeat twice.

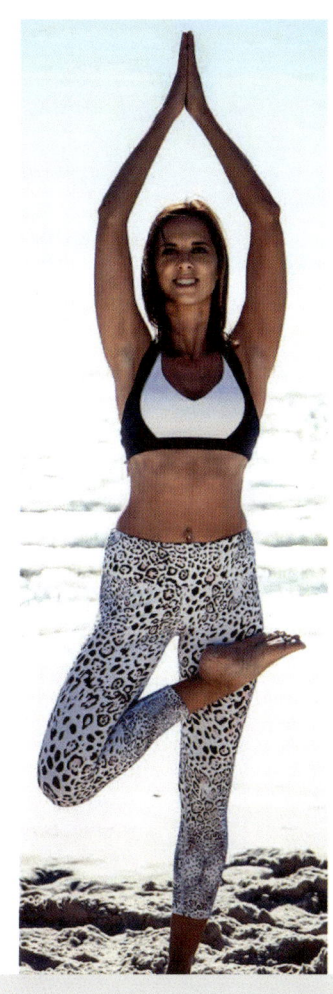

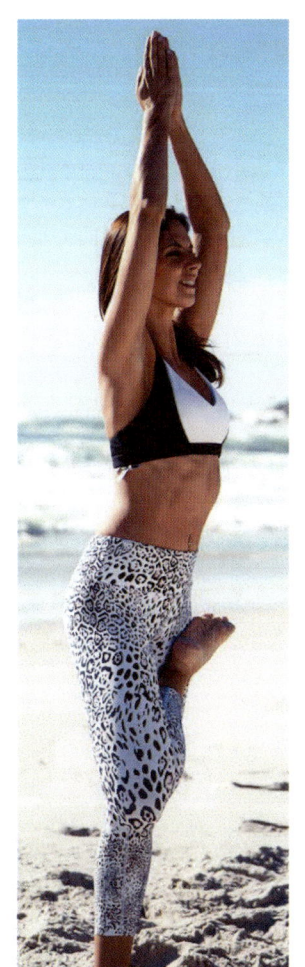

LONG AND NARROW

When you try this deeper hip flexor stretch, you will notice a few typical things might go wrong: your hips may tilt to one side if you don't lift the hips evenly, your shoulders want to come forward and your ribs and glutes will try to stick out (image on right)... because it's easier and **your body wants to do what's easier**. It's up to you to correct it. Remember to keep in check: KNEES, HIPS, RIBS, SHOULDERS!

To get into this stretch, stand strong on one leg. Hug the other knee to your chest and place the foot on the top of the hips. Bring foot up as high as possible into the opposite groin and gently unfold your knee towards the floor. If you can, bring both arms above your head.

Check you're all in line and hold for 30 seconds before you bring the knee back up to your chest and switch the legs: repeat the process. The aim is to imagine you are holding this stretch in a narrow gap between two walls.

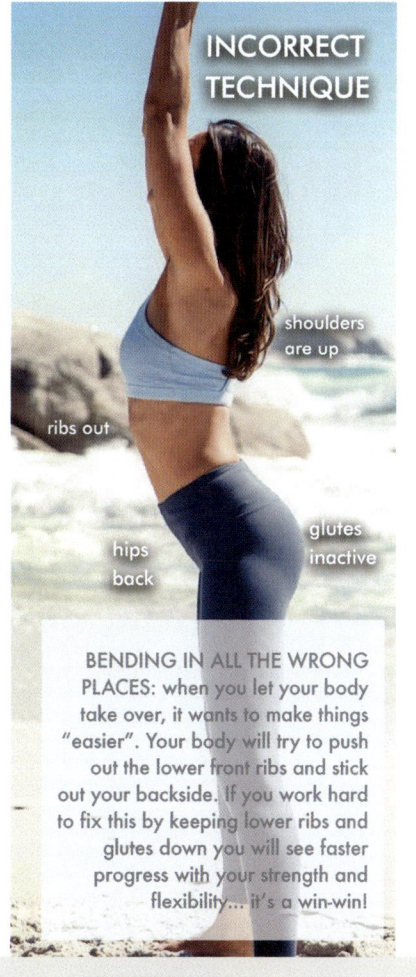

INCORRECT TECHNIQUE

shoulders are up

ribs out

hips back

glutes inactive

BENDING IN ALL THE WRONG PLACES: when you let your body take over, it wants to make things "easier". Your body will try to push out the lower front ribs and stick out your backside. If you work hard to fix this by keeping lower ribs and glutes down you will see faster progress with your strength and flexibility... it's a win-win!

© Jessica Zoo Ltd 2020 | BODY BEFORE SKILL Training Method   BBS Long & Strong - **BODY STRETCHES**

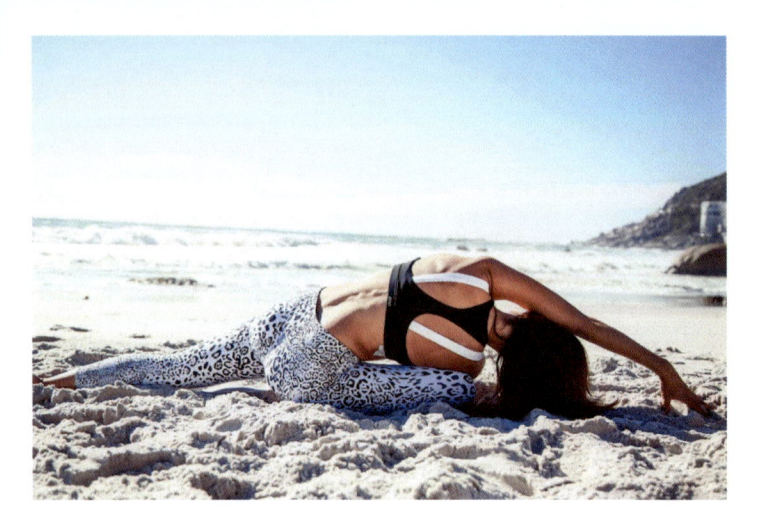

SPINE MOBILITY

The spine is the primary connection linking our brain to the rest of our body: increasing mobility is a tricky affair because if we push it too far, we can seriously create some damage. The most significant misunderstanding when it comes to back flexibility is that we can teach our spine to bend like a slinky toy: a recipe for disaster. Instead, we want to create space by lengthening and strengthening the areas around our vertebrae, so that it creates a strong but supple support system. Don't ever think of "bending" the spine, instead learn to mobilize it. One of the most incredible transformations through my own journey was combining yoga and Biokinetics training: I added 1.7cm to my standing height from creating more space and straightening my posture!

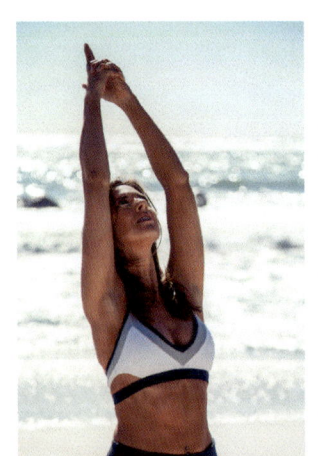

WARMING UP THE SPINE

The first step before you start any twisting or curling exercises with your spine is by warming up. Stand tall and strong, using all of your internal muscles around the vertebrae, including the core and back muscles to feel your spine in a long and strong position. Reach up with your hands but keep your shoulders down and front lower ribs in. Bring your hands back but still reaching for the ceiling and curve backwards to your ACTIVE end range. Slowly come back to centre, step feet wide and reach forwards into a straddle, curving your back so that it's concave. Repeat slowly for 2-3min.

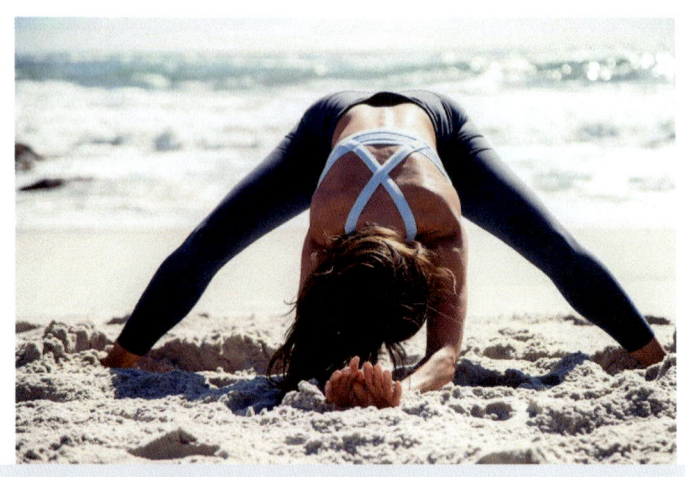

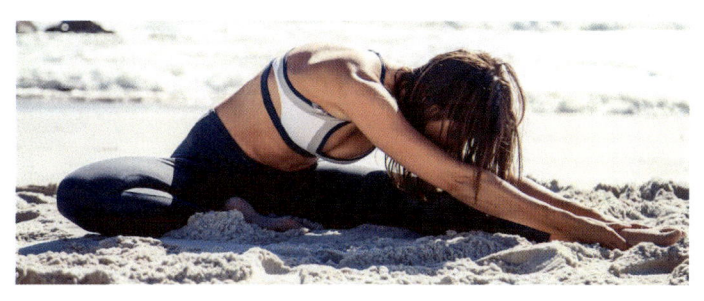

EXPLORE THE RANGE

When you're in your stretches, you usually want to keep the back straight to improve the length and flexibility of the targeted muscle. If you want to give your back a little more of a stretch, you can explore the movement by alternating between a straight back or making it concave. Whether you are rounded, straight, twisting, side or back bending: remember to visualize keeping your spine long and strong.

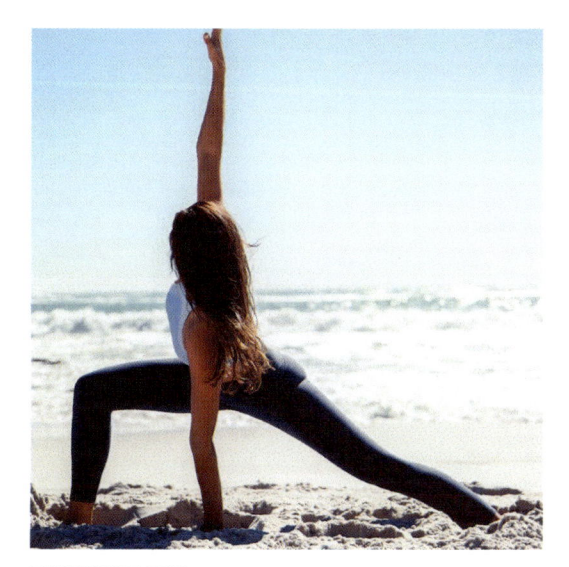

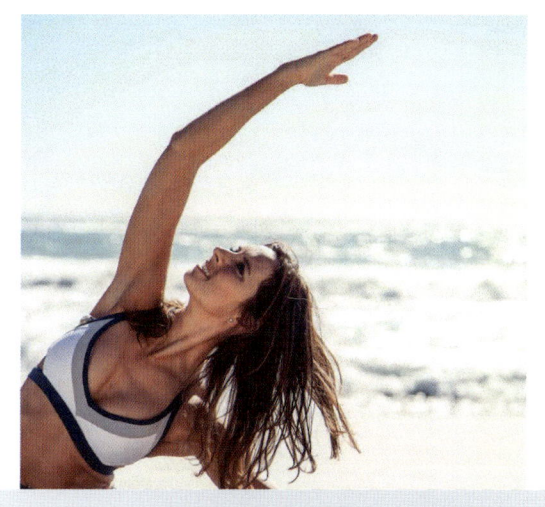

LET'S TWIST AGAIN

If you haven't already done so, this is a great place to try some of the twisting stretches that we have looked at in other sections. Before you perform more advanced backbends, make sure you've taken your spine through lateral torsion with long, strong twists.

This lunge twist is a great one to check if your spine is straight during a full side rotation. Reach the floor with both hands in your side lunge, with the front leg strong at 90 degrees. Side arm (same side as bent leg) goes up to the ceiling. Turn the chest whilst keeping the hips as square as possible. Aim to draw a straight line: hand-elbow-shoulder-shoulder-elbow-hand. Hold for 15 seconds before switching sides.

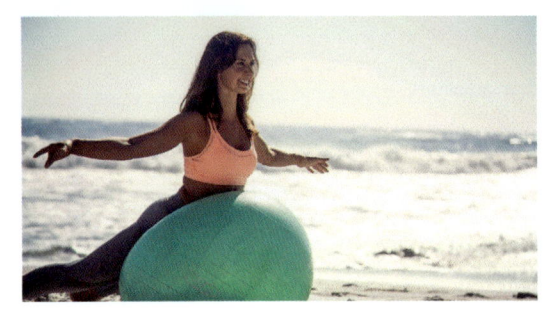

USING PROPS

Props such as a fitness ball, yoga blocks, straps, or even the sofa, a chair and some pillows - can be really helpful when you want to push yourself to new ranges of motion. A large exercise ball is a great back-bend buddy to help you develop back mobility.

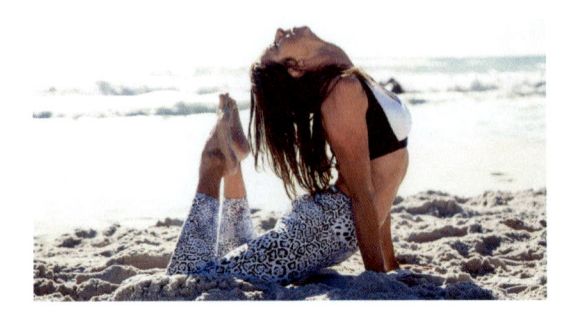

Hold each stretch for 20 seconds, breathing deeply into each gentle push.

Keep hips square, spine long and chest open at all times.

BE KIND TO YOUR SPINE:

listen to your body and only push yourself to where it allows you on the day.

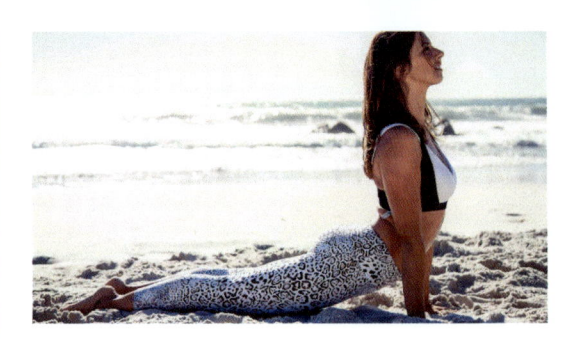

COBRA

The cobra is the first step into working your back bends: you can also start with a half-cobra with elbows on the ground. Start flat on the ground with hands by your sides. Make yourself as long as possible before pushing onto your arms and lifting into cobra.

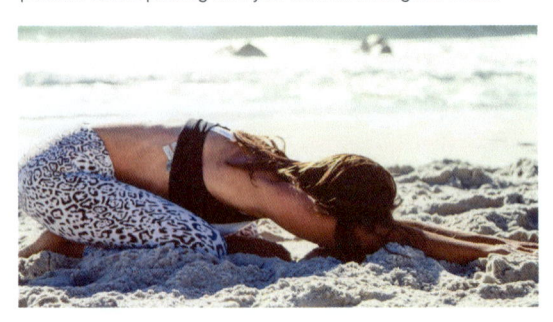

KING COBRA POSE

I'm still working on mine, so right now it's more of a "Prince" Cobra... From your cobra, the aim is to close the ring by getting your feet to your head. Push forward with your hips and support your spine by lifting. This also works hip flexor and quad flexibility.

CHILD'S POSE

After bending backwards a few times you might feel a bit dizzy or lightheaded. However **before leaning forward, kneel and sit upright**, stretching your arms up to the ceiling. Release the arms and go slowly/gently into a forward stretch like Child's pose.

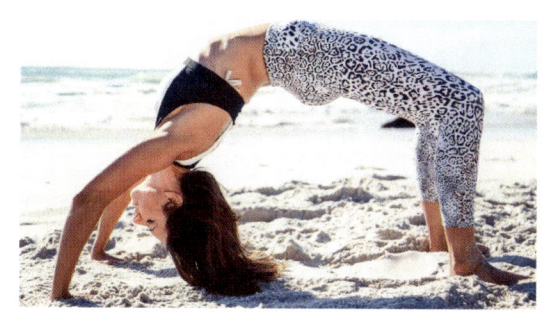

GETTING INTO A BRIDGE

The ability to perform a bridge correctly opens so many more realms of possibility of active flexibility skills, acrobatics and gymnastics. When you start practicing a bridge, it might look more like a "wheelbarrow" as you tend to collapse towards your feet.

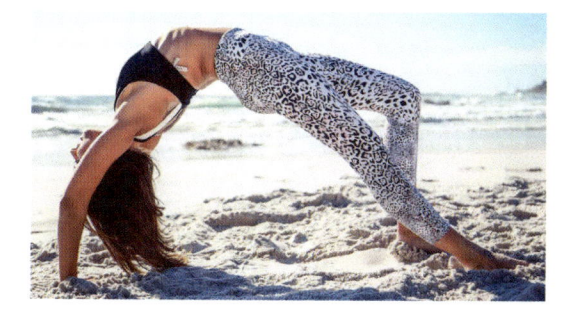

WALK THE BRIDGE

When you're in your bridge, start exploring more movement and strength by taking the weight off one foot at a time. This is a great place to develop your strength in holding the bridge, as well as your ability to move into and out of the skill.

Being able to do a bridge safely means you need to be assisted by a person you trust and that can guide you through the process.

If you've never done a bridge before, attend a class before you try this on your own.

If you already know how to do a bridge, you can work on your form and strength.

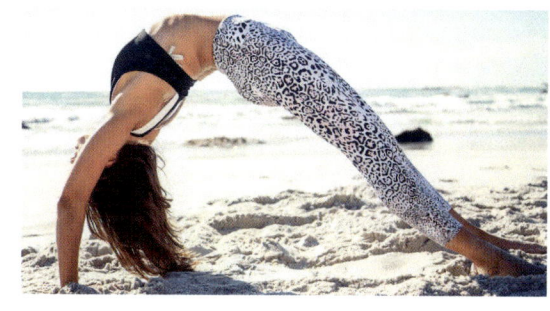

EXTENDED BRIDGE

A fully-formed bridge should lift up and away from the feet, looking like an upside-down check-mark. Your spine isn't the only area that needs attention: for a bridge you also need to work on hip, quad, shoulder and chest flexibility as well as arm strength. Mine is still work in progress while I work out shoulder restrictions.

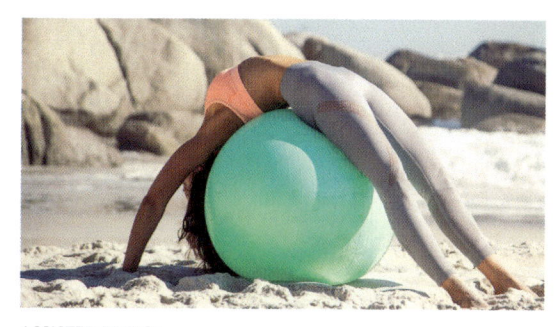

ASSISTED BRIDGE

This is great if you don't feel confident in your current strength, or you want to feel more secure in pushing up into a bridge. Using a fitness ball, a tumbling aid, or a stable, comfy chair will provide some assistance: a great way to develop a bridge more safely.

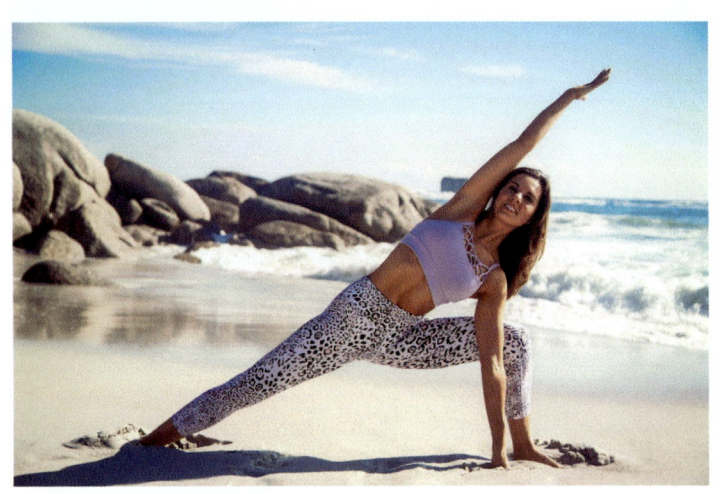

ACTIVE FLEXIBILITY

You might recall at the start of this guide, we mentioned that extensibility is an opposite quality of strength, but by working both together it can be extremely powerful to develop more impressive skills and helping you to prevent injury. Active flexibility is a way of developing ECCENTRIC STRENGTH (ie strength in extended ranges). Working on active flexibility skills separately is a must, otherwise you risk getting stuck in one of these common plateaus:

- **If you only work passive flexibility:** you can become supple but stay weak. This means your flexibility will be useless if you apply it to power skills such as gymnastics and holding shapes.
- **If you only work strength:** you will be stronger in your skills but will be limited by your range of motion.

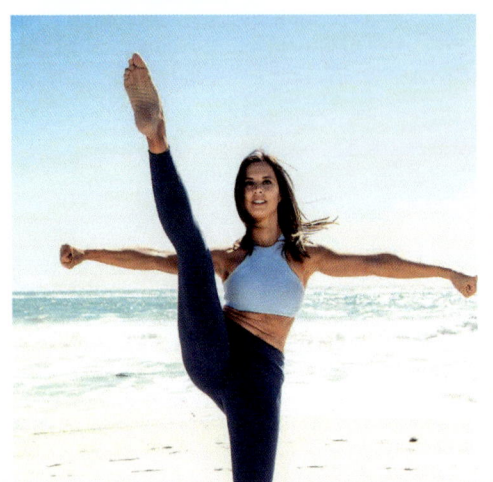

DYNAMIC VS STATIC TRAINING

There are two ways in which you can train active flexibility, both are needed to develop a good mix of power and stability:

DYNAMIC (left) is trained through ongoing movements. Start the move small and fast, in full control of your form. Using music is a great way to train this: use the BPM to direct your movement and hit the counts on the beat.

STATIC (right) using the same technique above, but we hold the shape statically in maximum active full range for as long as you can. Start holding for 1 second and work your way up.

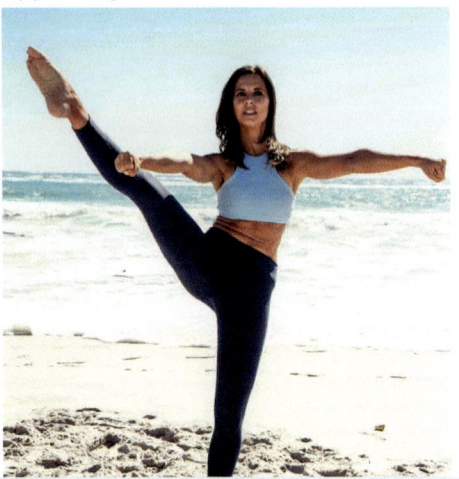

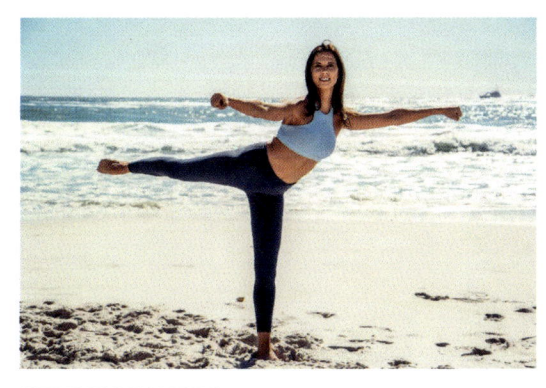

LIFTING VS COLLAPSING:

Let's play a game of "spot the difference" - what can you see that's different between the top picture and the lower picture, given that they showcase a similar range of flexibility in an arabesque? The main difference is that one is "lifted" while the other is "collapsing". One of the biggest misconceptions about flexibility is that muscles always need to be relaxed... it depends on which exercise. In active flexibility muscles should be **active and lengthening with an eccentric contraction** and you should be aiming to lift away from the standing foot, which is fully planted, wide and stable.

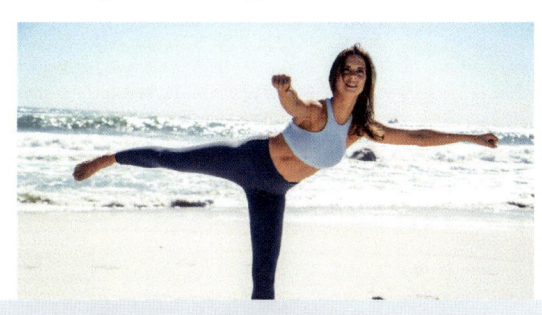

Hold each stretch for 20 seconds, breathing deeply into each gentle push.

Keep hips square, spine long and chest open at all times.

Be kind to your spine: it's not designed to curl and bend: listen to your body and only push yourself to where it allows you on the day.

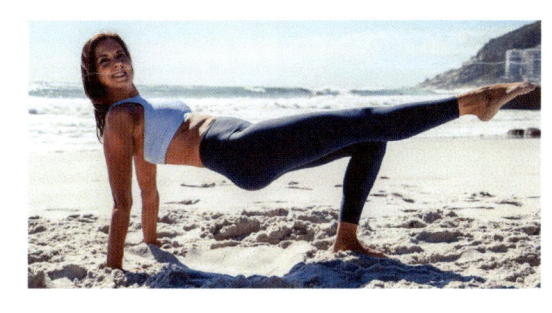

MOVE ON YOUR HANDS & FEET

Your hands and your feet also need to stretch in all directions, but they also need to be strong enough to support your weight. When you're on hands and feet, add a little bit of movement (like a gentle rotation or rocking) to strengthen the stability of your joints.

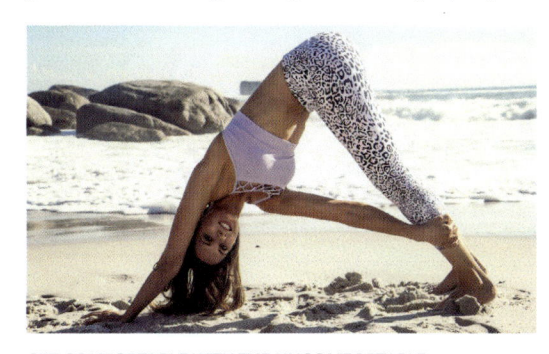

GET COMFORTABLE WITH THE UNCOMFORTABLE

Holding a stretch or a strength pose for a long time can become uncomfortable: that's normal! Your joints and muscles are getting used to holding strength at funny angles. The more you train and the more you become "comfortable with the uncomfortable" the stronger your joints and active flexibility.

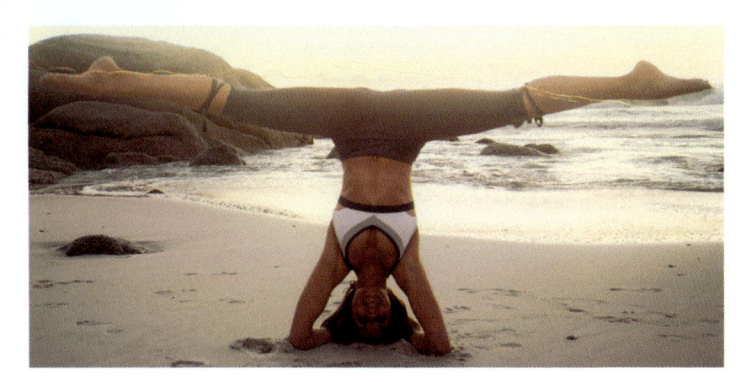

DEFYING GRAVITY

Another great way to stretch (and getting a great core and back workout at the same time) is stretching in a headstand position. Getting upside down for a few minutes a day is beneficial in so many ways and allows you to train the strength and flexibility of your stretches.

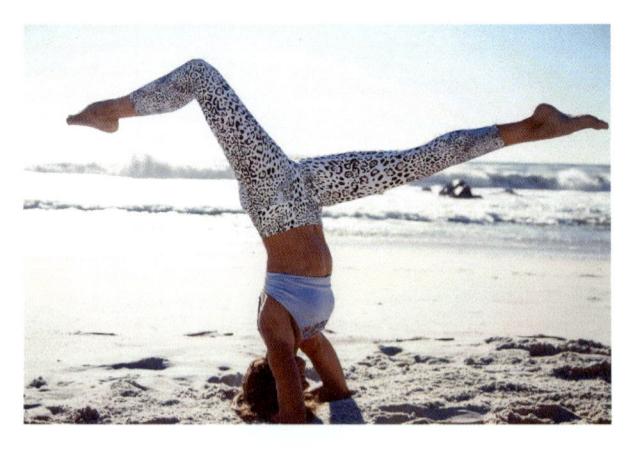

EXPLORE THE MOVEMENT
Once you have the strength and confidence to hold a headstand, explore the movements in a 3-dimensional way. You can also hold your static stretches and let gravity work its magic for about 20-30 seconds per stretch. **NOTE: If under 8 years of age, don't try this as your forearm bones are not strong enough yet.**

In your headstand, you want to *extend* the spine, not compress it! The head forms the third stability point of the "tripod" but the strength from the inversion comes from the outer edge of your forearm pressing strongly into the floor. Lift your shoulders strongly away from your ears and stretch your entire body up to the ceiling. Lower front ribs back, glutes lift up to your heels. You're creating a strong frame with your back and arms and lifting upwards all the time: pushing hard against your arms to create lift and stability.

STABLE BASE

Gravity can be conquered: go slow and steady by making sure you train your height slowly as you adjust your centre of gravity. Start off by training against a wall, and squeezing into a ball first: engage all the muscles and keep your spine straight. Once you're in your comfort zone you can slowly extend into a full vertical position. The trick is thinking long and strong. Push against the ground rather than collapsing.

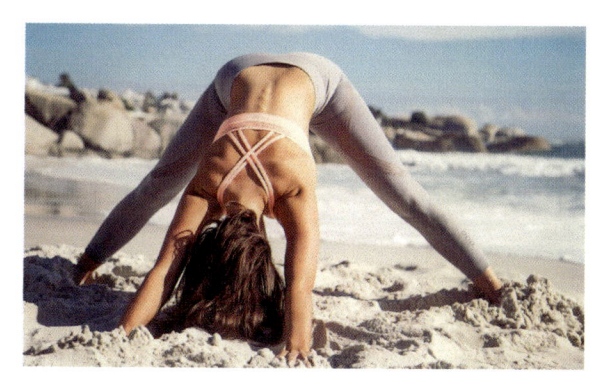

PUT YOUR BACK INTO IT

Before you try to get into a headstand (or in a handstand) the first step is learning to create strength and stability between your arms and your back. You can first practice in a down dog position or in a standing straddle stretch (pictured above). Shoulders are wide, strong, and away from the ears. You're attempting to make your arms as long as possible between the shoulder and the wrists. Lower front ribs back, hips in line with the feet, weight is on the feet. Arms are fully engaged and ready to take on the weight of your body. To see if you're handstand ready, try to go on your tiptoes or lifting one leg at a time. HEADSTAND & HANDSTAND tutorials are available in the BBS online workouts (ch.6).

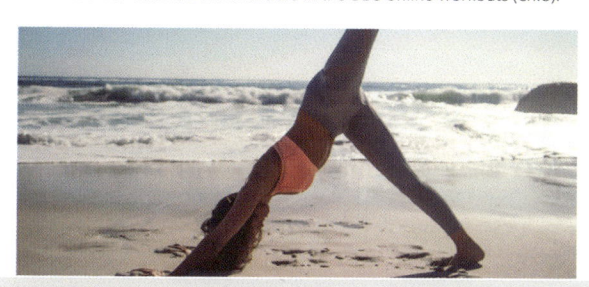

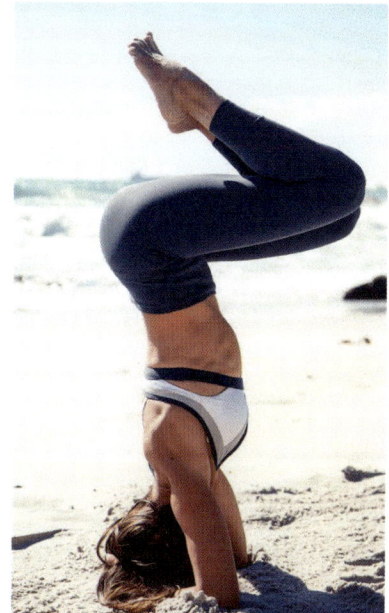

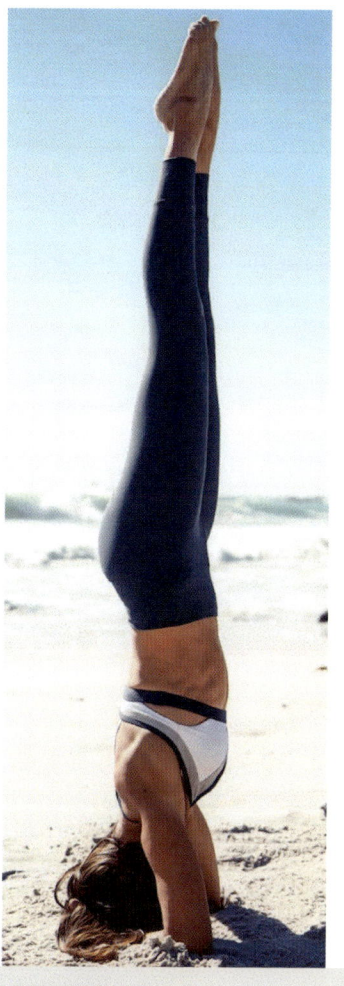

© Jessica Zoo Ltd 2020 | BODY BEFORE SKILL Training Method   BBS Long & Strong - **BODY STRETCHES**   41

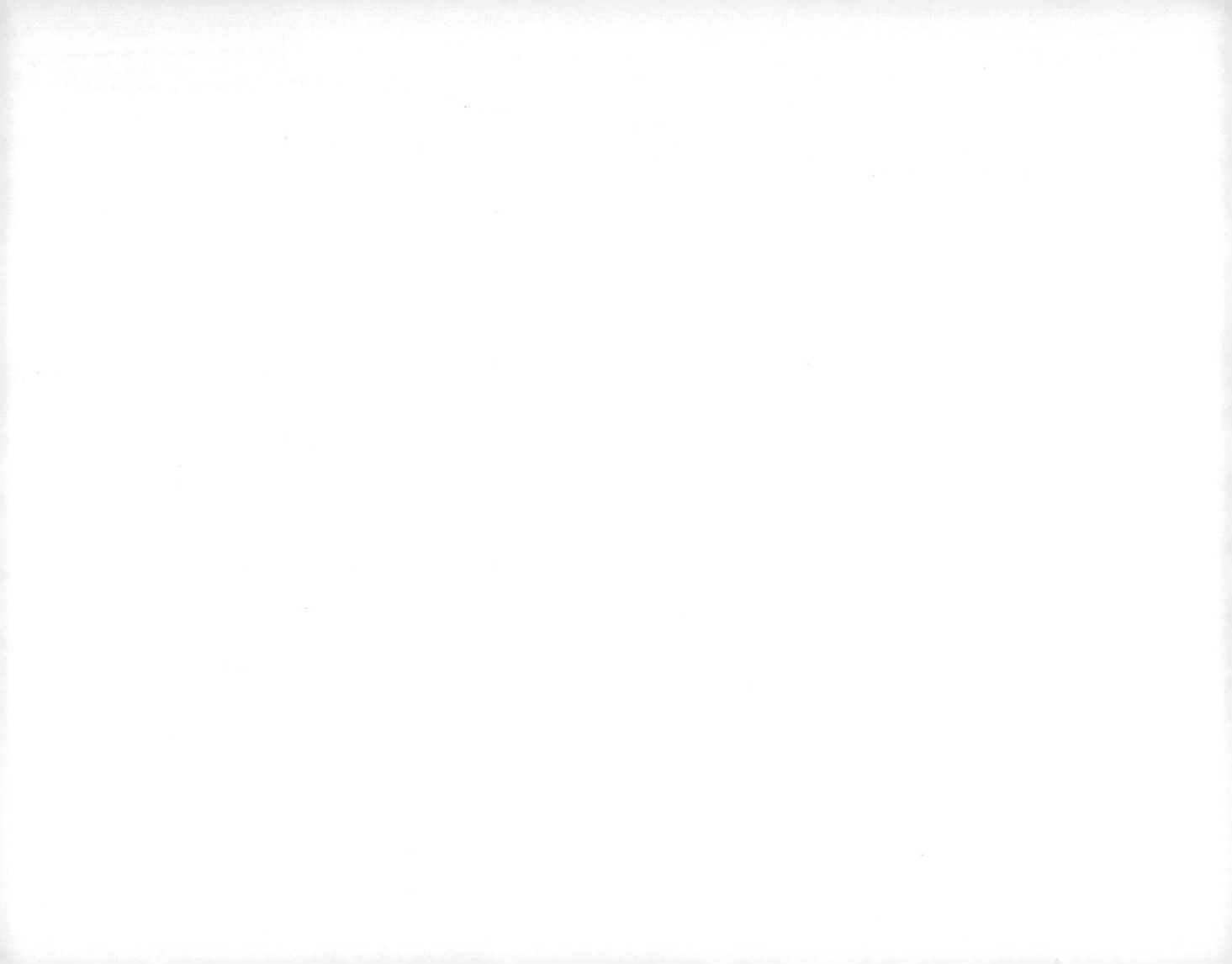

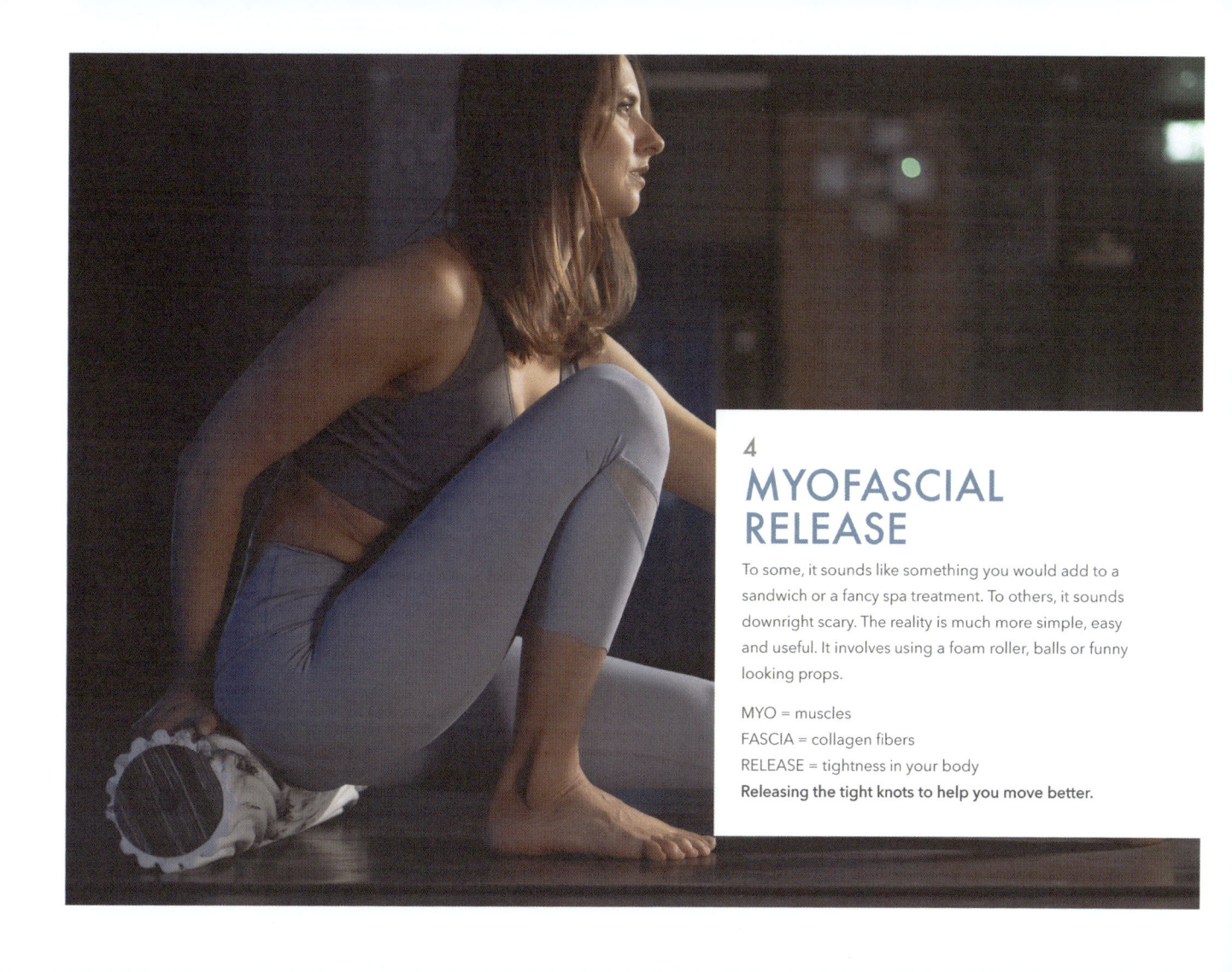

4
MYOFASCIAL RELEASE

To some, it sounds like something you would add to a sandwich or a fancy spa treatment. To others, it sounds downright scary. The reality is much more simple, easy and useful. It involves using a foam roller, balls or funny looking props.

MYO = muscles
FASCIA = collagen fibers
RELEASE = tightness in your body
Releasing the tight knots to help you move better.

WHY MYOFASCIAL RELEASE

Have you ever had a knot in your sweater? What happens when you pull? It just gets tighter. How many times have we tried to "stretch" a muscle that feels painful, only to find that it gets sorer? That's because you're *pulling* on it instead of *releasing it*.

A tight spot, also known as a knot, an adhesion or a trigger point: these are different ways of calling a small area of your body that's overworked. The muscle fibres, tendons and fascia can become tight and stiff (think of old chewing gum when you work on it for too long...). So you need to relax it, rehab and release it if you want to get rid of it.

Often, we see students struggle with flexibility and injury because they forget (or just don't know about) myofascial release. What you can do to help you **release knots or if you feel you have overstretched / recently injured an area:**

- Reduce stretching and increase myofascial release activity
- Use a foam roller or other massage props, using it on your entire body (not just your sore spots!) to iron out all the areas
- Self-massage using firm pressure and circular motions
- Rest and take a hot bath with Epsom salts
- Get a sports massage if the pain is obstinate, or see a physiotherapist if you feel something is not quite right
- Drink enough water - if your body is dehydrated it won't work properly
- Eat enough protein as part of a balanced diet

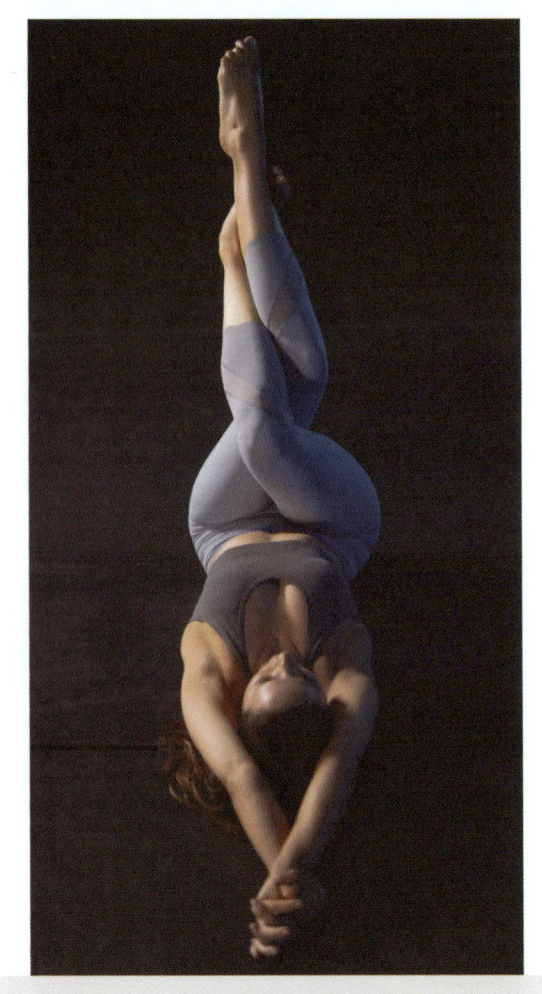

DON'T WAIT FOR THE PAIN

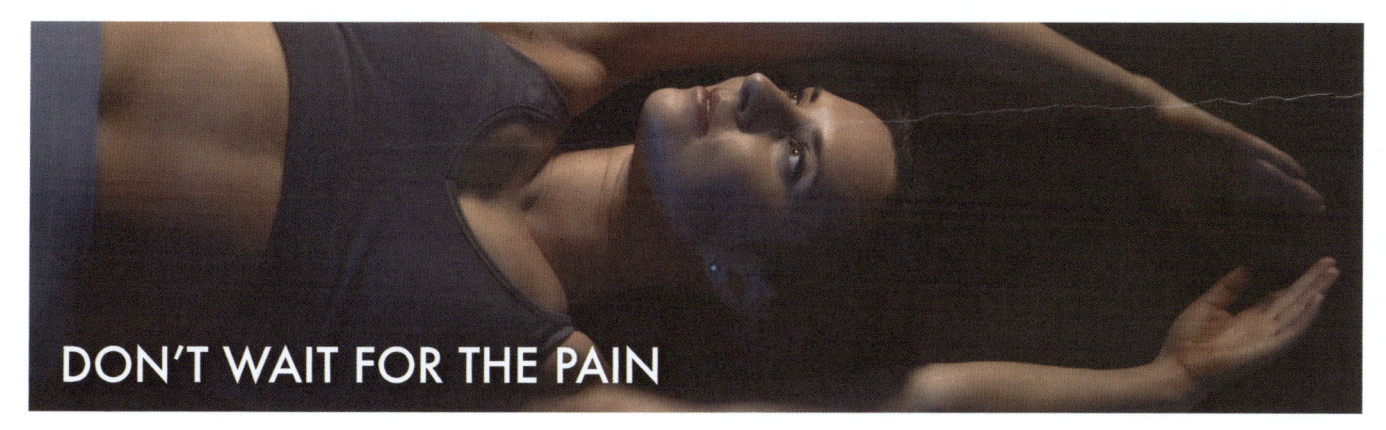

If you don't tune up your body in between workouts and practice, your risk of injury can multiply significantly. If you are injured, then your training was all for nothing. Your muscles are a complex biomechanical system working together as one. If one area is tight, it will pull more and create tension on the next muscle, and reduce its ability to work correctly. This might mean you can't perform a stretch or a skill you were able to before.

Pain is a clear sign that something is out of balance. When we over-train our bodies it decreases strength, power, flexibility and stability, but our immune system can also take a hit. This is why we tend to become ill when we're over-tired physically or mentally: our body is overworked. In addition, overtraining in one area can cause restrictions, sensitivity and tightness in your myofascial tissues. The pain usually originates from specific points within your trigger points. Myofascial release focuses on reducing pain by easing the tension and tightness in the trigger points.

Foam rolling, a hands-on form of myofascial release that you can do on your own, is the application of pressure to eliminate scar-tissue and soft-tissue adhesion by freeing up your fascia. This results in decreased muscle and joint pain, improved mobility, balance, posture, movement patterns and overall helps you achieve peak performance. Every muscle has its own optimal tension that allows your body to move the way it was intended to. When we work out and strain our body, it creates wastes such as acids and CO_2, as well as fighting the muscle stretch reflex that protects us against muscle tearing, or over lengthening.

WHEN & HOW TO FOAM ROLL

When is the best time to foam roll, and for how long? It depends entirely on your activity and why you're doing it.

GOAL	WHEN	TIME	AIM	HOW
For flexibility	before stretching a muscle group	2-3min per muscle group	To release tight spots that could be restricting your stretch potential	After your warm up and before any deep stretches, spend some time using your foam roller or ball to prepare the muscle groups you want to stretch.
As a warm up	before your training session	5-10min	To prepare your body to perform skills, to remove potential restrictions	Alternate stretching around 15 seconds and foam roll as necessary to help areas that may restrict you during your skills (especially front of the leg and shoulders).
For maintenance	as part of your cool-down or in between sessions	5-30+ min	To help break up any knotted tissues, while helping to pump new oxygen-rich blood to muscles, reduce soreness, return muscles to their original state	Alternate deep stretching and foam rolling as you would do in your flexibility training. Remember foam rolling for 5min every other day is better than one hour once a month. Spend as much time as you want.
For recovery	as prescribed	as prescribed	To help your body to recover: knowing your body and paying attention to changes in normal behaviour/ performance is key	If an area is sore, foam roll it and give it some TLC. Avoid stretching. Always consult a professional if you feel pain or something is wrong.

HOW TO ROLL (video demonstrations for each part of the body is available on the online video workouts).

- Focus on tender spots to alleviate knots that need to be worked through to help return muscles to their original tension.
- Use on the full body to help push new oxygen-rich blood through your muscles and help break up any acid build-up in them.
- Hold the roller on the tissue and "melt" onto the ball or roll until tightness reduces, for about 60 seconds.
- Breathe deep to relax, draw circles on the knot after the initial tightness is gone, to release more deeply.

5

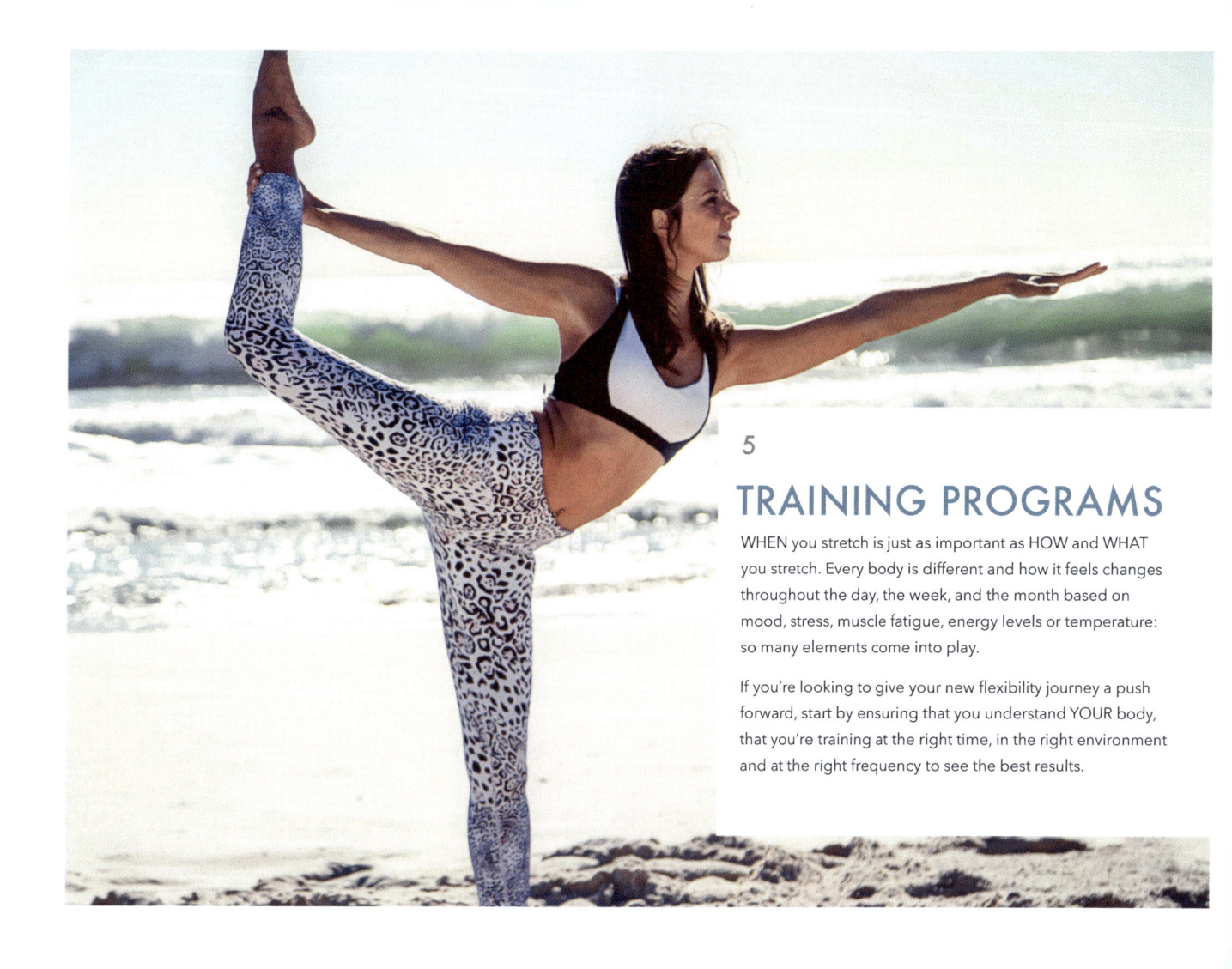

TRAINING PROGRAMS

WHEN you stretch is just as important as HOW and WHAT you stretch. Every body is different and how it feels changes throughout the day, the week, and the month based on mood, stress, muscle fatigue, energy levels or temperature: so many elements come into play.

If you're looking to give your new flexibility journey a push forward, start by ensuring that you understand YOUR body, that you're training at the right time, in the right environment and at the right frequency to see the best results.

STRUCTURE YOUR STRETCHING
Why do you need to think carefully about how, when and what you stretch?

What happens if you take an elastic out of the fridge, and yank it? Likely, it will snap. This is what you're doing to your body if you're pulling skills without warming up.

What happens if you take an elastic out of the drawer, and yank it apart with all your force? It will weaken and possibly tear. This is what you're doing to your body if you're performing skills before gradually stretching into your body's maximum active range.

What happens if you pull an elastic that has a kink or defect? It will continue stretching wonkily. This is what happens if you "scrunch" or stretch with bad technique or alignment.

What happens if you dangle a weight at the end of an elastic you've been stretching and pulling for about 15min? Likely, it will weaken and possibly tear. This is what you're doing to your body if you're training strength and power on muscles and joints you've been over-stretching during warm up.

What happens if you dangle a weight at the end of an elastic which is wide, strong and tough? It will stay strong, it won't move very much but if you yank it hard it will snap. This is what can happen to your muscles and joints if you avoid flexibility all-together: your body will be strong as long as it doesn't move beyond its limited range.

What happens if you dangle a weight at the end of an elastic that is thin, bendy and weak? It will overstretch so far that it will become weak, damaged, possibly torn in places and won't be able to lift the weight back up. This is what can happen if you're hyperflexible without training strength, or if you train flexibility using ballistic stretching.

WHAT'S THE BEST TYPE OF ELASTIC TO PULL? An elastic that is as strong as it is flexible. *An elastic that you get to know and understand how to handle safely!*

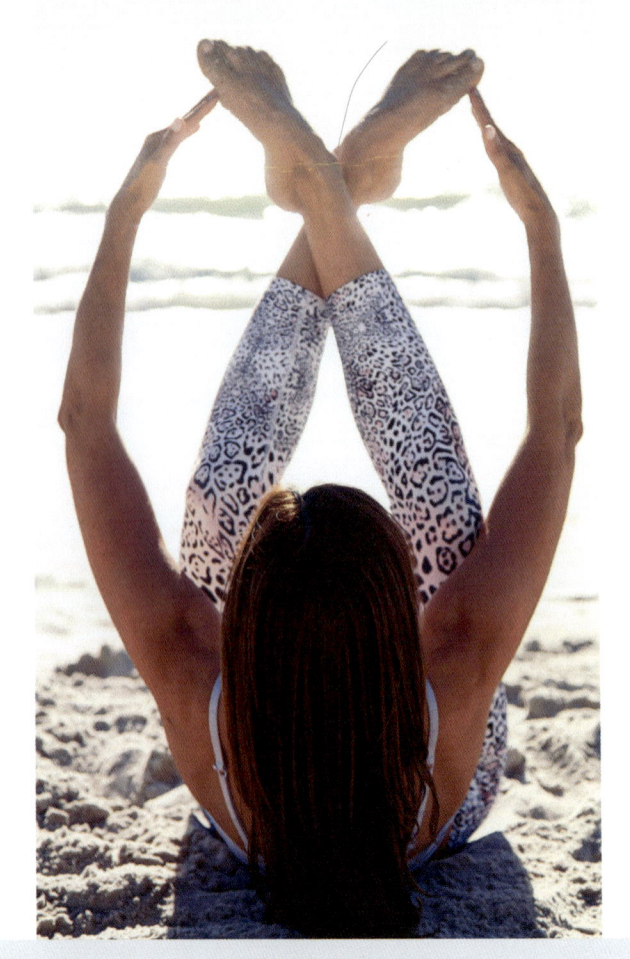

NAME:

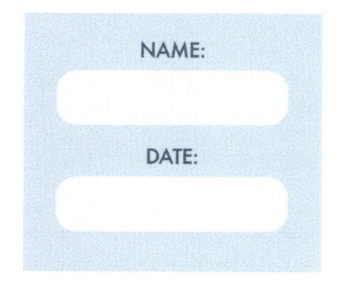

DATE:

COLOUR ACTIVITY

Every body is different. Get to know yours and the areas that need more of your attention.

Use a RED pencil to color in the areas that feel tight and in YELLOW the areas that feel weak.

Use the pressure of the pencil to color in harder for the areas that feel tighter or weaker. Print a few copies to keep track of the differences month to month!

If an area feels tight or weak, this is the area you should focus on. Both sides should be equally flexible too. Spend extra time working on your tight spots to bring your body to full flexibility.

BODY BEFORE SKILL™ KNOW YOUR BODY

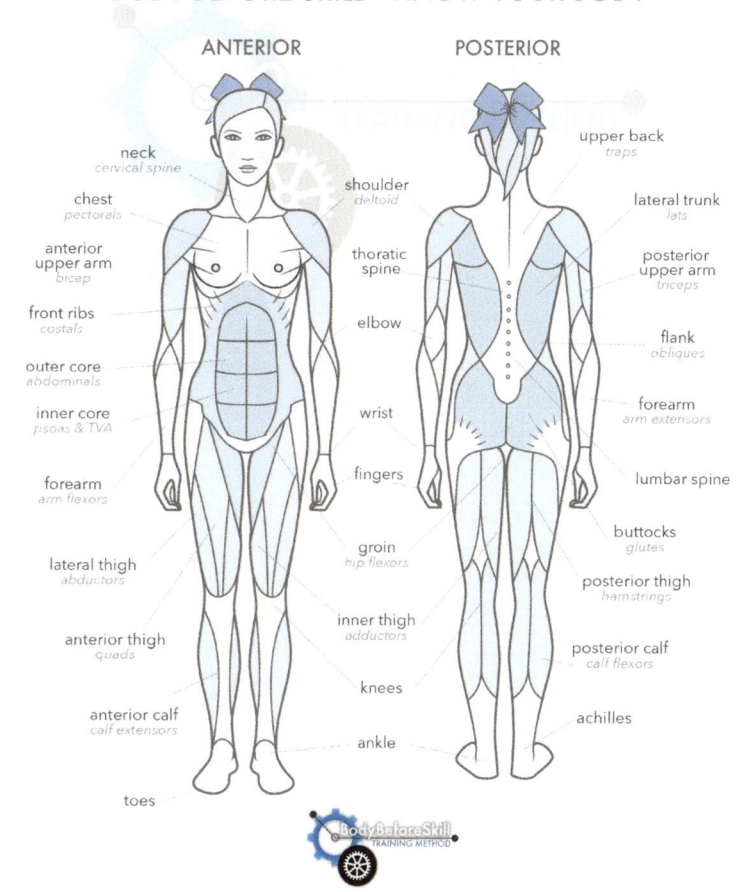

ANTERIOR

- neck — *cervical spine*
- chest — *pectorals*
- anterior upper arm — *bicep*
- front ribs — *costals*
- outer core — *abdominals*
- inner core — *psoas & TVA*
- forearm — *arm flexors*
- lateral thigh — *abductors*
- anterior thigh — *quads*
- anterior calf — *calf extensors*
- toes
- shoulder — *deltoid*
- thoratic spine
- elbow
- wrist
- fingers
- groin — *hip flexors*
- inner thigh — *adductors*
- knees
- ankle

POSTERIOR

- upper back — *traps*
- lateral trunk — *lats*
- posterior upper arm — *triceps*
- flank — *obliques*
- forearm — *arm extensors*
- lumbar spine
- buttocks — *glutes*
- posterior thigh — *hamstrings*
- posterior calf — *calf flexors*
- achilles

© Jessica Zoo Ltd 2020 | BODY BEFORE SKILL Training Method — BBS Long & Strong - **TRAINING PROGRAMS**

BEFORE / AT THE START OF A TRAINING SESSION

Based on the total time available before your training session, we highly recommend the following warm up structure to increase performance during the training session.

ACTIVITY	TIME	AIM	HOW
Cardio Warm Up	5-15min	Increase body temperature, activate muscle groups, awaken neuro-muscular system.	Bring your heart rate between 70-85BPM with a cardio activity
Dynamic Mobility & Stability Stretch	3-8min	Prepare maximum range of motion throughout the body. Strengthen (not weaken) muscle and joint power.	Go through standing dynamic stretches and include stability strength exercises
Skills Prep	3-5min	Go through all flexibility skills you need to perform during practice without pushing over current range	Warm up your skills without pushing beyond what your body is capable of doing.

AT THE END/AFTER A TRAINING SESSION

Based on your total time available at the start of your training session, work on restoring your body in the areas you have over-worked. Bring your body back into balance and this is a good time to push your flexibility.

ACTIVITY	TIME	AIM	HOW
Restore	5-10min	Reverse muscle over-use	Stretch all areas that have worked hard: especially chest, shoulders, hamstrings, glutes, any sore areas
Dynamic Mobility & Stability Stretch	3-8min	Push flexibility, prevent muscle stiffness	Use PNF, dynamic or partner stretch to stretch all areas of the body, and give your stretch skills a final good push
Re-fuel	at home	Replenish your glycogen levels and strength to your muscles with healthy carbohydrates.	For dinner, have some healthy carbs such as rice, sweet potatoes, corn, a healthy pasta, wholegrain bread, cauliflower.

AT HOME FLEXIBILITY: PICK YOUR GOAL

Depending on your goal, you will need a different stretch program. Rotate the phases during the GET FLEXY phases and the UPKEEP phases every 2-3 months to consolidate your strength at your current flexibility to avoid injury and build skill strength.

If you need to be on the "restore" cycle, follow with an UPKEEP month before starting a GET FLEXY cycle.

Avoid "GET FLEXY" style of program during competition season to reduce the risk of injury. Stop GET FLEXY at least 2 weeks before your first event, performance or a competition. You can start again once competition season is over and you're safe from over-working.

	COMMITMENT	AIM	Warm Up	PREPARE	WORK IT	OTHER
GET FLEXY	50min sessions 4-5 times per week + stretch after practice	Increase range of movement of your entire body and achieve new flexibility skills	Spend 5-15 minutes warming up: cardio and dynamic warm up.	Spend 30min stretching your entire body with 3D movement: using a mix of dynamic, static and PNF techniques	Work on your flexibility skills using static stretching and PNF method. Spend 2min on each skill.	Avoid any strength training, cardio or practice in the 18 hours that follow your "GET FLEXY" stretch session.
RESTORE	30min sessions 3-4 times per week + stretch after practice or workout	Restore your body after weakness, injury or stiffness.	Spend 5 minutes warming up focusing on gentle, controlled movement in the area that feels sore.	Spend 20min focusing on the area using gentle dynamic movement and static stretching. Feeling should be sore, not painful. See a doctor if you feel ANY pain.	Hold main static stretches for 2minutes each. Use foam roller or ball to work on areas that feel sore.	Epsom salt baths, myofascial release, sports massage or physiotherapy session if the niggles are persistent.
UPKEEP	35min session once a week + stretch after practice or workout	Keep your flexibility where it is, strengthen body tolerance at current level of flexibility	Spend 5 minutes warming up using a dynamic warm up routine.	Spend 20min giving yourself an all-round body stretch	Challenge yourself by holding the flexibility skill in the air, wobble board or handstand. Get creative and build strength with your mobility.	Increase strength and stability conditioning. Use foam roller or ball to work on areas that feel sore.

FLEXIBILITY TRACKER

Month: Year:

My 3 Goals This Month:

Day	Time spent stretching	What feels tight?	What feels weak?	Achievements
1				
2				
3				
4				
5				
6				
7				
8				
9				
10				
11				
12				
13				
14				
15				
16				
17				
18				
19				
20				
21				
22				
23				
24				
25				
26				
27				
28				
29				
30				
31				

YOUR L&S ACCESS CODE FOR BBS ONLINE STUDIO:

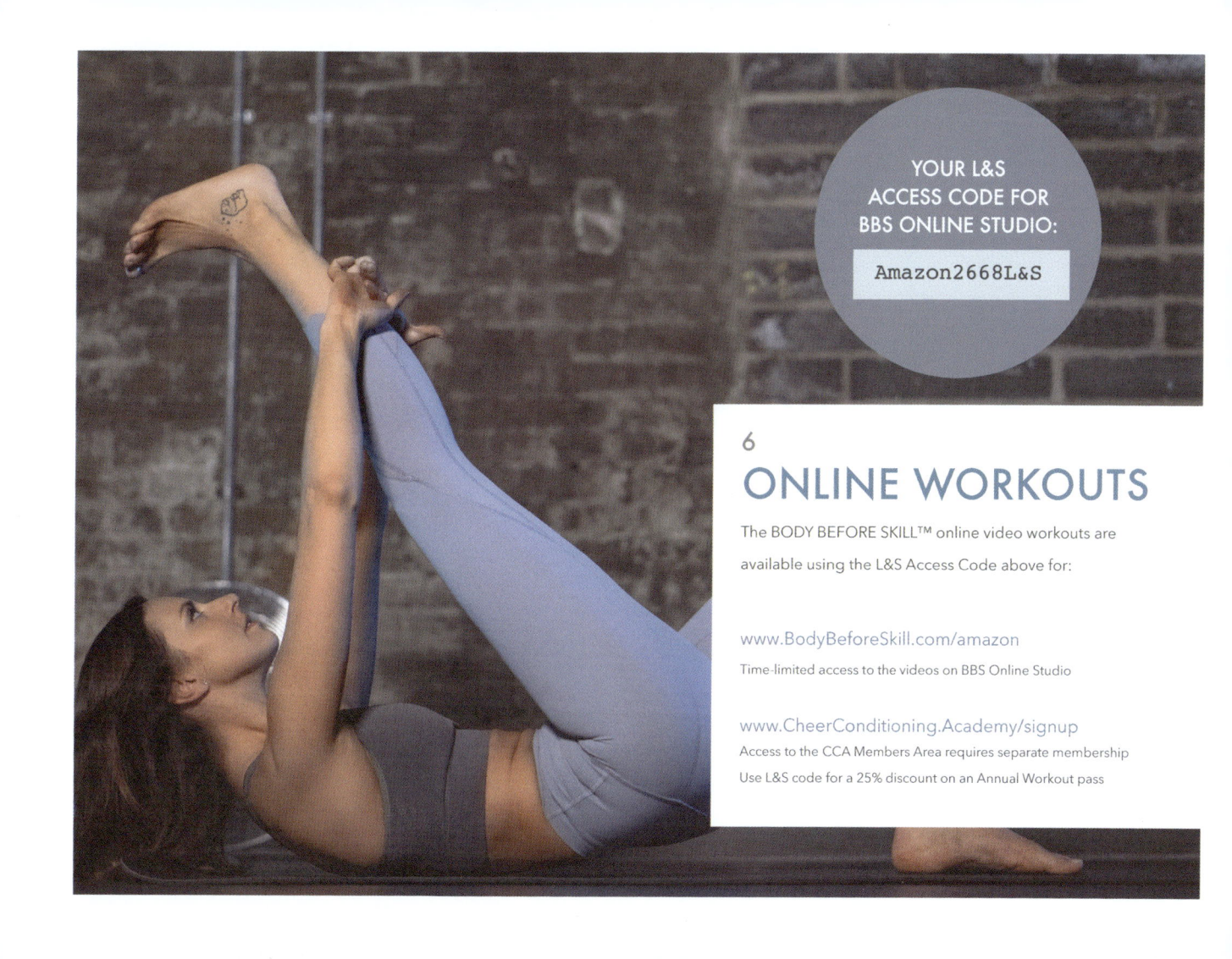

Amazon2668L&S

6
ONLINE WORKOUTS

The BODY BEFORE SKILL™ online video workouts are available using the L&S Access Code above for:

www.BodyBeforeSkill.com/amazon

Time-limited access to the videos on BBS Online Studio

www.CheerConditioning.Academy/signup

Access to the CCA Members Area requires separate membership
Use L&S code for a 25% discount on an Annual Workout pass

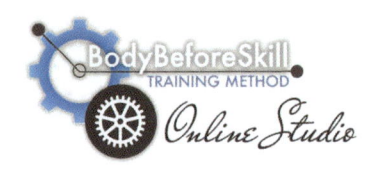

WELCOME TO YOUR BBS STUDIO

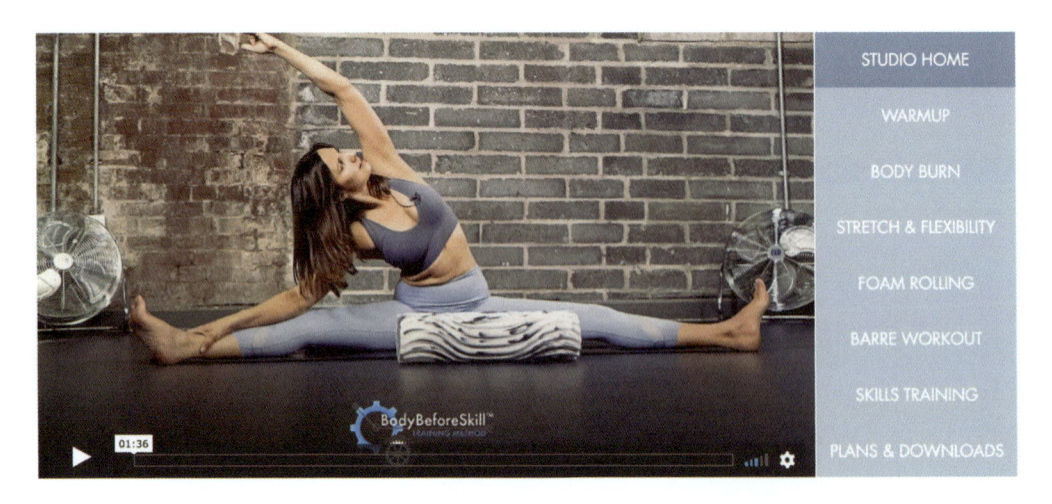

STUDIO HOME

WARMUP

BODY BURN

STRETCH & FLEXIBILITY

FOAM ROLLING

BARRE WORKOUT

SKILLS TRAINING

PLANS & DOWNLOADS

The BBS Online Studio features playlists, workouts and classes focusing on a blend of techniques that focus on movement optimisation, flexibility and development of lean body mass.

Each workout is carefully crafted to blend the joy of movement, music and exercise science for an optimal online training experience. Each section comes with its own recommendations and equipment suggestions. Explore to get started and have a look at the PLANS & DOWNLOADS.

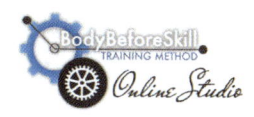

HOW TO USE THE PLAYLISTS

PLAYLIST	DESCRIPTION	USE VIDEOS FOR YOUR WARM UP	TRAINING SESSION	COOL DOWN
WARMUP	Individual tracks designed for dynamic warmup and awareness.	START YOUR TRAINING HERE with 1 or 2 videos	N/A	N/A
BODY BURN	Individual tracks designed as a cardio boost or for endurance training. Use individually or as a playlist.	N/A	Use 1+ tracks as you wish, but always BEFORE your Stretch & Flexibility	N/A
STRETCH & FLEXIBILITY	Sequences targeting lengthening of specific body areas. Use individually or as a playlist.	N/A	Use 3-6 tracks as needed if you're doing a stretch/ flexibility session	Use 1-2 tracks if using as a cool down
FOAM ROLLING	Sequences targeting myofascial release of specific body areas	N/A	Use before/in between stretching & flexibility to release tensions / knots	Focus on your BACK
BARRE WORKOUT	Full 1 hour classes aimed at active flexibility, stability, endurance & developing lean muscle mass	Warmup, workout & cool down INCLUDED - full 60min class BARRE will help train/develop active flexibility.		
SKILLS TRAINING	Individual skills broken down into technique and training exercises.	N/A	Use as needed, as part of your training session	N/A
PLANS & DOWNLOADS	Download BBS Long & Strong e-guide. Quick review of workout plans, training guidelines and playlists.	Read the BBS Long & Strong book BEFORE you start your training. The BBS Training Method is a blended way of training through knowledge and awareness.		

CHEERCONDITIONING ACADEMY
Members Area

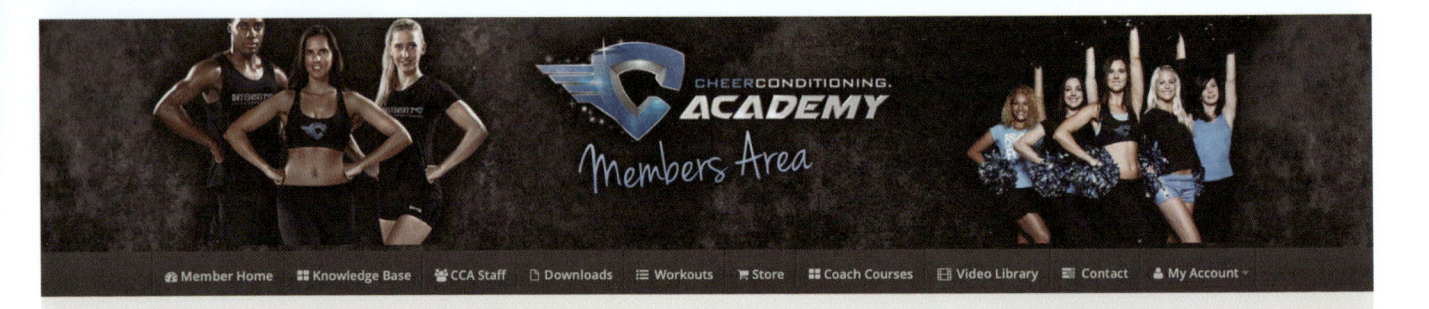

| Member Home | Knowledge Base | CCA Staff | Downloads | Workouts | Store | Coach Courses | Video Library | Contact | My Account |

Hello Jessica!

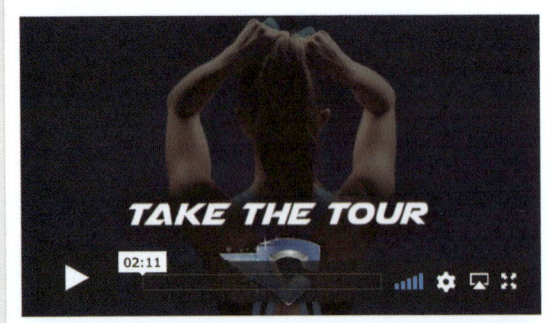

TAKE THE TOUR
02:11

LET'S GET STARTED!!

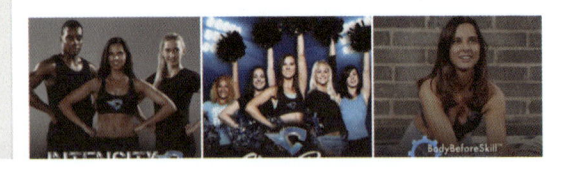

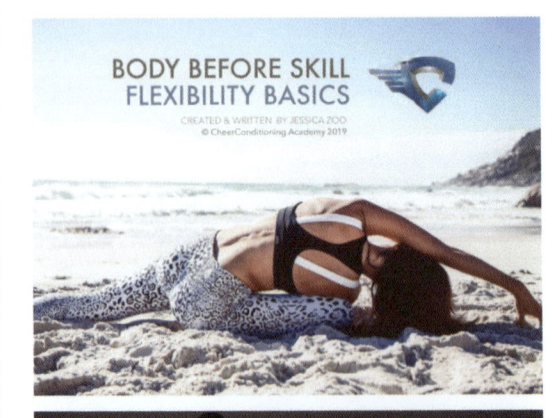

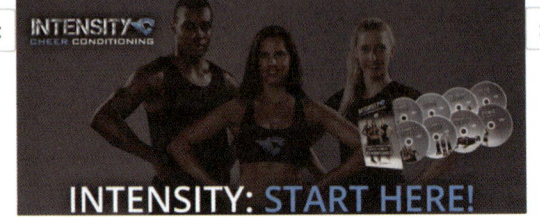

BODY BEFORE SKILL FLEXIBILITY BASICS
CREATED & WRITTEN BY JESSICA ZOO
© CheerConditioning Academy 2019

INTENSITY CHEER CONDITIONING
INTENSITY: START HERE!

HOW TO USE THE VIDEOS

To access the training videos, you will need to sign up using your *L&S Access Code* to sign up to the BBS Online Studio on www.BodyBeforeSkill.com/amazon You can also access BBS training videos on the CheerConditioning.Academy (CCA) Members Area, which is a separate platform and membership. Your *L&S Access Code* also serves as a 25% discount voucher on CCA workouts.

- DOWNLOAD THE 30-Day FLEXIBILITY OPTIMISATION PLAN
- Always start your training session with one or more warm up tracks
- Apply the techniques you have learned in this guide to maximize results
- Make sure you have your equipment before you start
- Watch and listen to the demonstrations carefully
- Listen to your body and stop if you feel any pain
- Consult a medical professional or therapist if you feel unsure/unwell/in pain

SUGGESTED EQUIPMENT

Yoga or pilates mat
Ballet shoes or non-slip socks
Barre, sturdy chair or kitchen counter
Pilates ball
Bands
Light weights 0.5kg-3.0kg

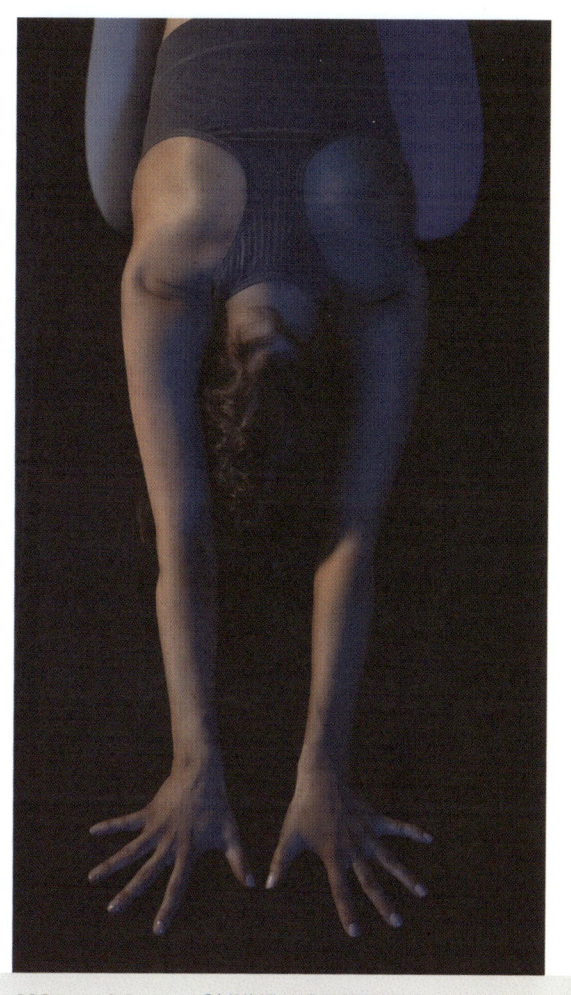

NOW IT'S YOUR TURN TO GET LONG & STRONG!

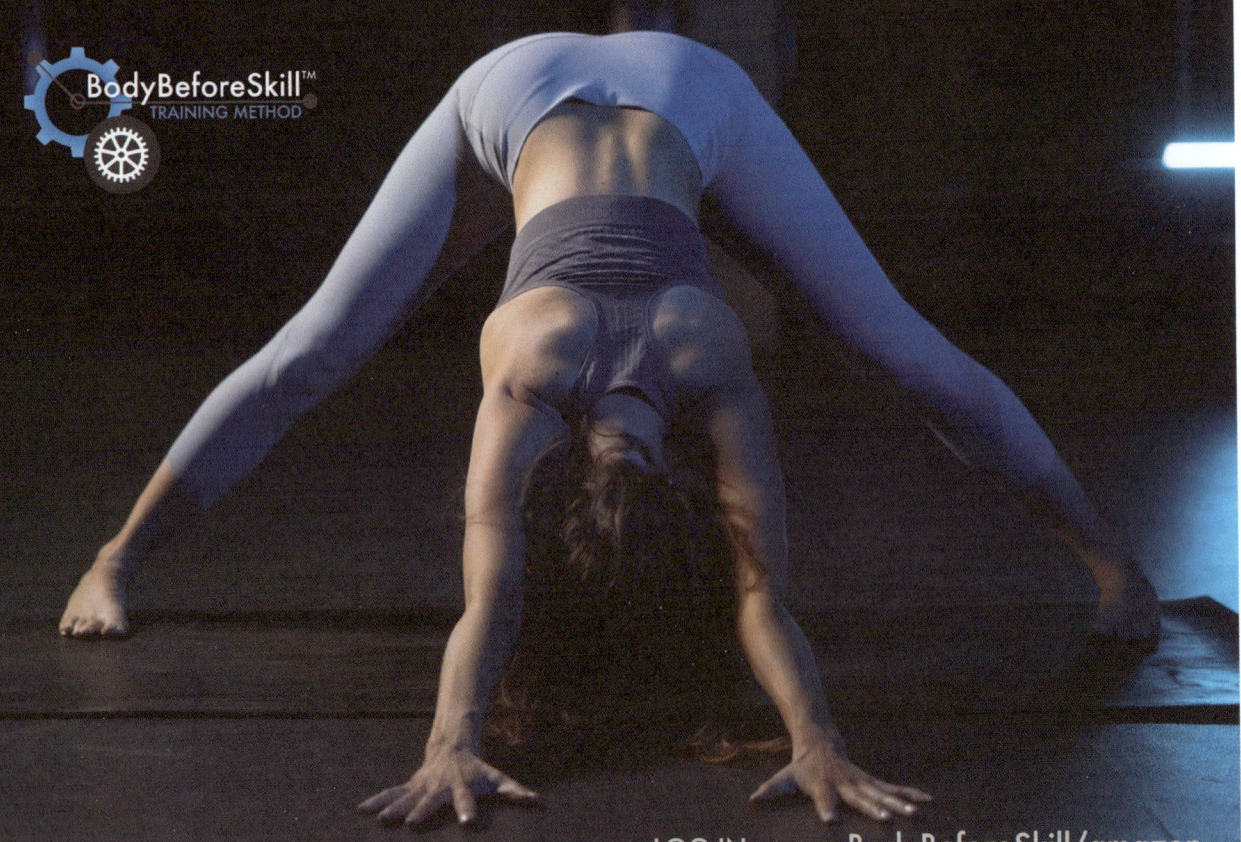

BodyBeforeSkill™
TRAINING METHOD

LOG IN: www.BodyBeforeSkill/amazon